The conservation of teeth

The conservation of teeth

J. D. ECCLES PHD, FDSRCS

Emeritus Professor of Conservative Dentistry, Dental School,
Welsh National School of Medicine, Cardiff

R. M. GREEN BDS, PHD

Reader in Conservative Dentistry, Dental School,
Welsh National School of Medicine, Cardiff

SECOND EDITION

BLACKWELL SCIENTIFIC PUBLICATIONS

OXFORD LONDON EDINBURGH BOSTON MELBOURNE

© 1973, 1983 by
Blackwell Scientific Publications
Editorial offices:
Osney Mead, Oxford, OX2 0EL
8 John Street, London, WC1N 2ES
9 Forrest Road, Edinburgh, EH1 2QH
52 Beacon Street, Boston
   Massachusetts 02108, USA
99 Barry Street, Carlton
   Victoria 3053, Australia

First published 1973
Second edition 1983

Printed in Great Britain by
the Alden Press, Oxford
and bound by
Green St Bindery,
Oxford

DISTRIBUTORS

USA
   Blackwell Mosby Book Distributors
   11830 Westline Industrial Drive
   St Louis, Missouri 63141

Canada
   Blackwell Mosby Book Distributors
   120 Melford Drive, Scarborough
   Ontario, M1B 2X4

Australia
   Blackwell Scientific Book Distributors
   31 Advantage Road, Highett
   Victoria 3190

British Library
Cataloguing in Publication Data

Eccles, J.D.
   The conservation of teeth.—2nd ed.
   1. Dentistry
   I. Title   II. Green, R.M.
   617.6′01   RK501
   ISBN 0-632-01136-X

Contents

Preface to second edition

Since the first edition was completed there have been a number of changes in the pattern of dental disease and in the practice of conservative dentistry. The prevalence of dental caries in the United Kingdom has been declining, more dentists are incorporating prevention as an integral part of their practices and low-seated four-handed dentistry has become firmly established. It would appear that the attention given to prevention and operating methods in the first edition was fully justified. These chapters have been altered in detail but not in concept. The age distribution of the population has altered slightly with more people retaining their teeth into old age and so we have started to give some consideration to the restorative problems of the older patient.

This edition includes a number of techniques which have become established since 1972 but the chapter headings have been kept essentially the same except for Chapter 9. With the decline in importance of the cast gold inlay and the increasing use of full-coverage crowns it was decided to expand this chapter to include all anterior and posterior full-coverage crowns. A description of laboratory procedures has been omitted since textbooks have become available which deal with these very satisfactorily. Chapter 15 has also been omitted.

In the first edition it was hinted that traditional fully extended restorations were not always indicated. In this edition it is made clear that a good preventive attitude by the patient is of vital importance and that cavity size should be reduced and tooth tissue conserved whenever practicable. The essentials of occlusion have been discussed more fully, but detailed consideration of this topic must be left to the specialist texts.

Preface to first edition

Although a number of ancient civilisations practised reparative and restorative dentistry on a very small scale, the period of Pierre Fauchard (1678–1761) can be considered to be the beginning of dentistry as a healing art. Conservative dentistry developed as a main branch of this art. Considerable contributions were made to its progress by many dentists and in particular by Dr. G.V. Black (1836–1915) of the USA. Textbooks on conservative dentistry, or operative dentistry as it is sometimes called, during the period up to the middle of the twentieth century reflected the attitudes and interests of the dentists of the period and concentrated largely on restorative techniques. Very high technical standards were sometimes achieved. Although research also developed this was of necessity primarily pure research and most clinical techniques were carried out on an empirical basis.

Prior to the Second World War there were signs of a change in outlook and this developed rapidly after the War and led to radical changes in thought and gradual improvements in the practice of dentistry. These changes were mainly in three directions, the introduction of new techniques, a change in attitudes, and the further development of research. Advances in techniques were perhaps the most obvious of the changes and included the development of high-speed cutting equipment, used in conjunction with the washed field technique and high-volume suction, and the development of new operating methods. But if the changes in techniques were the most obvious, the changes in attitudes were the most important. These included the realisation of the role which dentistry must play in the dental health of the community rather than in the care of individuals; the appreciation of the limitations of reparative techniques and the fact that, without successful prevention, it would be impossible to achieve a state of dental health in the community; the concept of total patient care rather than the restoration of individual teeth; and the development of efficient working methods in an attempt to make dental care available to more people and to lighten the arduous work of the dentist. The development of research was of considerable importance; the accent changed to applied research, taking advantage of the basic research which had been and was being carried out, but in spite of this there is still much empiricism in the teaching and practice of dentistry. Research into dental materials continued to develop and became orientated more in biological and clinical directions.

The writers believe that these changes in the practice of dentistry, and particularly their application to conservative dentistry, require a reorientation of the textbooks on this subject. The present work is an attempt to meet this. It aims to take into consideration changes in education which emphasise ideas rather than facts. The student of dentistry who understands principles and is capable of creative thinking will be better equipped to meet the changes of the future than the student who has only learned facts. While the book is designed primarily for dental students, it is hoped that some of the thoughts and views expressed will be stimulating to general practitioners.

The authors understand the objectives of conservative dentistry to be the same as those of dentistry as a whole, namely the achievement and maintenance of the oral health of the community. It is only in the nature of its contribution to oral health that conservative dentistry differs from other branches. The World Health Organisation has defined health as a state of complete physical, mental and social well-being, and not merely the absence of disease and disability.

Oral health is the contribution of the mouth and teeth to health. To be more specific, oral health aims at bringing about and maintaining a state where the appearance of the mouth and teeth is as good as the patient's tissues will allow; where the function of the mouth in mastication and speech is as good as can be obtained, and where there is an absence of pain and discomfort. The form of the teeth and oral tissues should be such that reasonable efforts on the part of the patient can maintain them in a healthy condition, free from dental caries and periodontal disease. Conservative dentistry deals mainly with the hard tissues of the teeth which may be affected by dental caries. It is also concerned with the relationships of the adjacent teeth, the treatment of abnormalities of the hard dental tissues, the prevention and treatment of trauma to the teeth and the welfare of the adjacent periodontal tissues. Prevention must play a major role in the maintenance of oral health. It is therefore essential for the dentist to educate individual patients in diet control, oral hygiene and other preventive measures they can practise, as well as to educate the community in communal measures of prevention.

By tradition in this country, conservative dentistry for children under the age of 10 or 12 is included in the discipline of child dental health and for this reason will not be discussed. Endodontics, crowns, bridges, impact injuries to the teeth and the science of dental materials will not be considered since excellent texts already exist in these fields.

Acknowledgements

We should like to acknowledge the valuable assistance of Mr Mel Davies, who read the proofs of Chapters 9 and 10 and gave much helpful advice, Dr David Adams who brought us up to date with the precautions needed to treat patients who have suffered from viral hepatitis, and Mr Reg Day who advised us on porcelain crown aesthetics. We were most fortunate to continue to have the help of Mr Robert Starr and Mrs Patricia Ware who were responsible for the photography and artwork respectively and who continued the high standard they achieved in the first edition. We are grateful to Mrs Eve Baxter for typing the new parts of the manuscript and to Mrs Wendy Petschnyk for secretarial support. The Editor of the *British Dental Journal* kindly gave her permission to reproduce Fig. 9.25 b & c. To Professor B.E.D. Cooke, Dean of the Dental School, Welsh National School of Medicine, Cardiff, we again owe our thanks for the use of photographic, illustration and typing facilities.

Chapter 1
Teeth and their environment

An architect, designing a building, does not consider it in isolation. He takes into account the effects that it will have on adjacent buildings and those on the opposite side of the street. Equally, he considers the way in which existing or planned structures will affect his building. He explores the availability of services and a whole range of environmental and social problems. In addition he needs to understand the properties of the constructional materials he is using and the engineering and aesthetic problems involved. He must also keep abreast of advances in his field.

Similarly, the dentist cannot consider restoration of an individual tooth in isolation. He needs to take into account the effect of his proposed restoration on the adjacent and the opposing teeth and their effects upon it. He has to understand the factors present in the oral environment of his patients. He must appreciate the clinical and biological properties of the materials that he uses and have an understanding of the engineering and aesthetic problems involved. Finally the dentist must be aware of the varied social requirements of his patients.

Before considering the conservation of teeth, therefore, it is essential for the student to have a basic knowledge of the teeth and their environment. Firstly he must be familiar with the normal appearance, structure and function of the teeth and the surrounding tissues. Secondly he should have a knowledge of the aetiology of dental caries and other conditions which lead to the loss of tooth substance. Thirdly he must appreciate the effects which these have on the dental tissues. Finally he must understand the biological effects of the operative procedures and restorative materials which he uses. It will be taken for granted that the student has a knowledge of the normal structure and function of teeth. In the space available, it will not be possible to give more than a brief appreciation of the pathological features but it is hoped nevertheless that this will allow the student to begin to understand the problems involved whilst encouraging and indeed obliging him to delve further for himself.

I

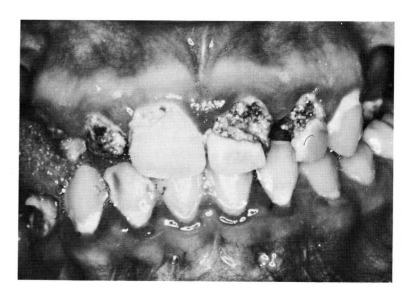

Fig. 1.1 Extensive caries in a 16 year old girl. Early 'white' carious lesions are visible particularly on the upper left and lower right canines.

Dental caries

Dental caries is a disease which commences on the surfaces of the teeth which are exposed in the mouth. It results in the gradual destruction of the hard tissues of the crown of the tooth (Fig. 1.1), and following gingival recession may also affect the exposed portions of the roots. If untreated it progresses to the dental pulp and may destroy the entire crown of the tooth. It leads ultimately to pain, loss of masticatory function, inflammation of the gingival tissues, abscess formation, deterioration in the patient's appearance and related social effects. The disease is widespread in civilised countries, where few people escape its attack.

Dental caries involves the destruction of the hard tissues by the action, initially, of acid-producing bacteria on the surface of the tooth. It is, in its early stages, a slow sub-surface demineralisation of the dental enamel. This is progressive and continues through the enamel, across the enamel–dentine junction and into dentine. The demineralisation is accompanied, particularly in the dentine, by some degree of proteolysis. In the older patient where some gingival recession has occurred carious lesions can develop in the cementum and dentine of the exposed root of the tooth.

Any tooth present in the oral cavity acquires an intimate covering of salivary deposits, bacteria and by-products of bacterial metabolism (Fig. 1.2). This complex material is called dental plaque. It adheres to the smooth enamel surface and also collects in the deep grooves and fissures. It continues to accumulate unless

Fig. 1.2 Dental plaque.
(*upper*) Author's mouth (RMG) after three days without oral hygiene. The normal diet was supplemented with four ounces of boiled sweets each day and these were sucked slowly. The plaque was stained with gentian violet and the mouth rinsed.
(*lower*) As above but after normal tooth brushing for one minute.

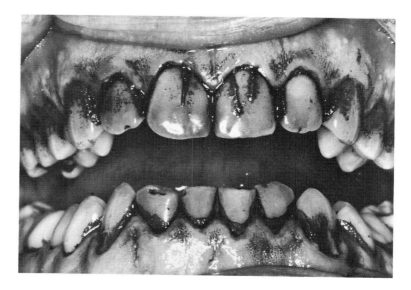

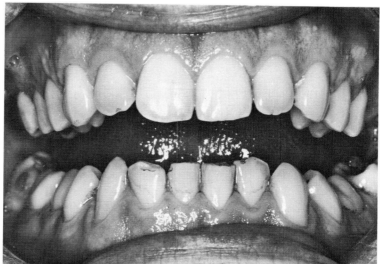

removed by oral hygiene procedures or, to a limited extent, by the action of fibrous foods during mastication. Unfortunately neither of these has much effect on the plaque in the deep fissures. Dental plaque constitutes a very specialised micro-environment within the oral cavity. The frequent intake of refined carbohydrate enables the monosaccharides and disaccharides to permeate into the plaque where they are either metabolised directly or built up into intracellular and extracellular polysaccharide reserves by the

3   *Teeth and their environment*

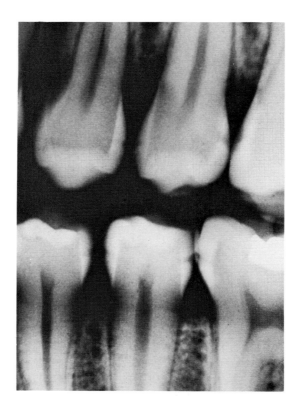

Fig. 1.3 Bitewing radiograph showing small radiolucent dark areas on approximal surfaces indicating early caries of the enamel.

bacteria. The intracellular polysaccharides act as an immediately available energy reserve for the bacteria at times when free monosaccharides and disaccharides are not available. The extracellular polysaccharides serve two functions; one part, the polyfructans, appears to form a labile energy reserve in much the same way as the intracellular polysaccharides, whilst the remainder, the polyglucans, forms a remarkably stable slimy gelatinous mass which helps to locate the bacteria and their metabolic waste products against the tooth surface.

As the bacteria continue their normal metabolic processes within the plaque organic acid waste products accumulate. The presence of these acids within the gelatinous matrix leads, in turn, to the characteristic sub-surface demineralisation of the early carious lesion. On naked eye examination such a lesion on a smooth tooth surface appears as a white porous area softer than the healthy enamel and with a lower light reflectance giving it a chalky appearance (Fig. 1.1). After a time, if the caries does not progress too rapidly, it absorbs stains and subsequently varies in colour

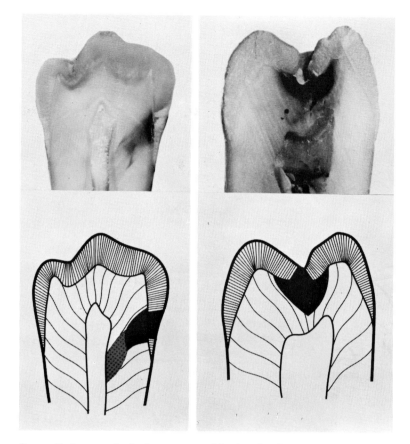

Fig 1.4 Spread of caries from (*left*) a smooth surface lesion and (*right*) a fissure lesion. Caries is shown diagrammatically in black. Note the general tendency for spread along the paths of the enamel prisms and dentinal tubules, with lateral spread at the enamel–dentine junction. The shaded section corresponds to the area of modified dentine between the carious lesion and the pulp.

from light to dark brown or black. Such early lesions on approximal surfaces can be conveniently demonstrated by radiographic examination when they appear as small radiolucent dark areas clearly seen in bitewing radiographs (Fig. 1.3). If plaque continues to be retained on the affected surface the carious lesion will progress and cavities will be produced. However, if the environment can be changed to avoid the accumulation of plaque, or the diet altered, or the tooth surface made more resistant, the lesion can be arrested at this stage.

In caries in fissures the pattern is similar, except the surface of the tooth is folded on itself so the early white stage of the lesion is seldom seen clinically. The first stage which can normally be identified is either slight cavitation, which can be detected by a probe, or a dark discoloration of the fissure. The carious lesion as it develops within the enamel appears to spread most rapidly along the path of the enamel prisms with relatively little lateral spread.

However, once the lesion penetrates to the enamel–dentine junction it spreads more rapidly and in a lateral as well as in a direct course along anatomical pathways. This general tendency of dental caries to follow the path of anatomical features within the tooth leads to two distributions depending upon whether the caries starts from the linear area of a fissure or from a wider area on a smooth surface. The two patterns of spread are shown in Fig. 1.4 and these must be borne in mind in the treatment of established caries.

So long as a lesion is confined within the enamel there is the possibility that it can be arrested and remineralised by a change in the environment. At this stage there is little or no positive reparative response within the dentine or pulp. However, once a lesion has penetrated into the dentine the odontoblasts respond to the stimulus by laying down calcified tissue within the pulp space and in the tubules. Prior to restoration the survival of the pulp in a vital state depends on the balance between the speed of development of the carious lesion and the rate of deposition of secondary dentine. If the carious lesion comes into contact with the pulp the latter becomes infected and inflamed. This leads, over a period, to irreversible changes and finally to pulpal necrosis. The detailed histological sequelae in the enamel, dentine and pulp following carious attacks are described in textbooks of dental pathology.

COMMON SITES FOR CARIES

The micro-environment at the tooth surface is very important in the occurrence of caries. Equally, the anatomical features of the tooth influence considerably the micro-environment on different parts of the tooth surface. Plaque forms on all surfaces of the tooth but it becomes firmly established only on those areas of the tooth protected from the action of fibrous foods and tooth brushing. Caries is generally associated with such areas of undisturbed plaque formation and these can be readily recognised. They are:

● *The pits and fissures* The narrow clefts at the base of pits and fissures form an ideal protected environment for bacterial growth. Plaque accumulates easily and caries is common although the physical bulk of the plaque is not great.
● *The areas of contact* between the approximal surfaces of the teeth. Around the contact area is a protected space in which bacteria can establish themselves and proliferate. This in turn results in the formation of an undisturbed plaque and frequently caries is produced.

- *The gingival third* of the buccal and lingual surfaces of most teeth. This is another relatively sheltered area for bacterial growth where caries may occur. Below the line of maximum convexity of the tooth surface, heavy deposits of plaque tend to form as it is protected by the curvature of the tooth from the effects of the passage of fibrous food and from the cursory oral hygiene measures practised by many people. However, plaque in this area can be removed by careful brushing thus distinguishing it from the situation in the fissures and contact areas.

For many years it has been common practice to refer to these areas of the tooth as 'caries susceptible' whilst referring to the remainder of the tooth surface as either 'caries resistant' or 'self-cleansing'. The implications of this terminology are not supported by the findings of modern research. There is little evidence to suggest any variation in caries susceptibility of the dental enamel in the different areas of the tooth surface. It has also been shown that, even under extremely favourable conditions, the action of fibrous foods is not sufficient to remove plaque completely from the whole of any tooth surface. Regular and active oral hygiene procedures are essential if plaque accumulation is to be effectively controlled. It would appear more reasonable to regard the tooth surface as being divided into areas which are readily cleansable and other areas which are not. It is clear that the three basic areas associated with the occurrence of caries come to varying degrees within the latter category.

Tooth surface loss

In addition to dental caries there are three major conditions, abrasion, attrition and erosion, which may result in the loss of hard tooth tissue and whose control is important in the conservation of teeth. They differ from caries in that the loss is essentially from the tooth surface and plaque is not involved. Some degree of tooth surface loss can be considered as normal wear and tear; it is only when this becomes excessive and threatens the function, appearance or comfort of the dentition that it may require treatment. Early recognition of excessive tooth surface loss is necessary to enable preventive measures to be instituted.

Abrasion is the result of abnormal wear of the teeth by foreign bodies. The typical abrasion cavity, caused by forceful horizontal brushing along the necks of the teeth, is associated with gingival recession and appears as a polished groove at the cervical margins of the teeth on their buccal sides (Fig. 1.5). The lesion primarily affects the cementum and dentine of the root whilst the harder enamel is less affected. Toothbrush abrasion is more pronounced on prominent teeth such as canines or teeth adjacent to an edentulous area.

Attrition results from the wear caused by one tooth on another and primarily affects occlusal surfaces, incisal edges and the contacting surfaces of upper and lower anterior teeth. By itself, it rarely requires treatment but may do so if it is associated with erosion.

Erosion is the loss of hard tooth substance resulting from the action of chemicals, principally acid. The most common cause is the excessive drinking of acid beverages and consumption of citrus fruit; some common beverages and fruit juices have a pH between 2 and 3. The lesions occur primarily in the enamel which appears abnormally smooth, shiny and rounded with the loss of surface features. If they are not treated or arrested the lesions progress into the dentine and appear as wide, shallow depressions (Fig. 1.6). A second cause of erosion is industrial and is found in workers in those industries where acid aerosols are regularly encountered in the atmosphere. This type of erosion affects the parts of the upper and lower anterior teeth which are exposed, either during speech or when the lips are at rest. A third source of acid is the habitual regurgitation of gastric contents which produces lesions on occlusal surfaces, incisal edges and the palatal surfaces of upper teeth. Abrasion and attrition often contribute to the damage caused by erosion.

The surrounding and supporting structures

The restoration of a tooth which has been damaged by caries is of limited value unless the surrounding and supporting structures of the tooth are healthy enough to allow it to remain in the mouth as a useful functional unit. In addition, the restoration must be executed in such a way as to cause the minimum damage to these structures in the short term and in the long term.

Few people have completely healthy gingivae; the majority of mouths show some degree of inflammation of the marginal gingivae. It is highly desirable that this should be reduced to a minimum before a restoration is placed. Operative procedures should be carried out with minimum trauma in case this tips the balance further towards disease. Marginal gingivitis is associated with the microbial activity of the dental plaque and, while this

Fig. 1.5 Abrasion at the necks of lower teeth in a 53 year old man, associated with horizontal brushing.

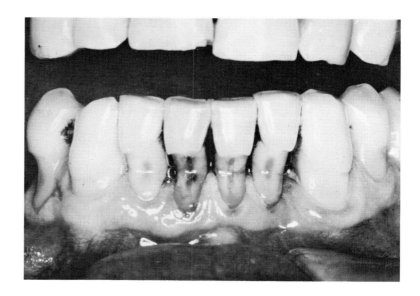

Fig. 1.6 Erosion on the labial surfaces of lower anterior teeth in a 38 year old woman, associated with a diet containing much citrus fuit.

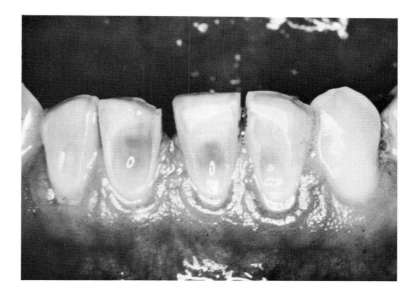

differs from the mechanism of dental caries, a reduction in plaque will lead to a reduction in caries and to improved gingival health. Plaque must be removed at least once a day in order to prevent gingival disease and the build-up of a sufficient thickness to cause caries.

The presence of a restoration encourages the formation of

Fig. 1.7 Bitewing radiograph showing loss of alveolar bone between the molar teeth associated with poor approximal contour and an excess of amalgam at the gingival margin of the mesio-occlusal restoration in the second molar.

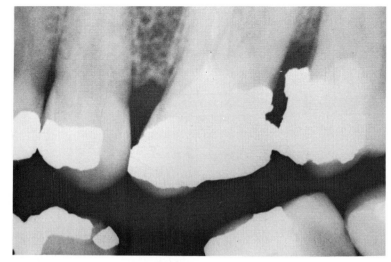

Fig. 1.8 Sixteen year old amalgam restoration showing food packing in the embrasure (*left*) resulting from a fractured marginal ridge (*right*).

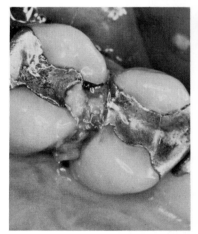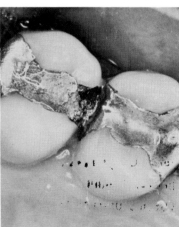

plaque and any surface roughness or marginal defect allows a nucleus of plaque to remain after cleaning (Fig. 1.7). Chronic marginal gingivitis is frequently present around sub-gingival restorations and secondary caries may commence in marginal deficiencies.

Relationship between adjacent teeth

An understanding of the relationship between adjacent teeth is important in making a satisfactory restoration. In a complete arch teeth usually touch their adjacent neighbours at the contact areas.

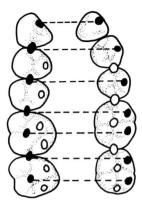

Fig. 1.9 Occlusal surfaces of upper and lower posterior teeth showing areas of contact in centric occlusion (centric stops). The black areas show where the buccal cusps of the lower teeth (*right*) occlude with the marginal ridges and fossae of the upper teeth (*left*). The white outlines show the occlusion between the palatal cusps of the upper teeth and the marginal ridges and fossae of the lower.

Immediately below the contact area in young patients is the gingival col which terminates in buccal and lingual peaks. In older patients, or where a pathological condition is present, there may be an interdental space below the contact area.

Laterally, the tooth surface curves from the contact area on to the buccal and lingual surfaces. Occlusally, the marginal ridge has a protective action. If the contact area is not restored, or is poorly contoured in a restoration, food may be forced inter-dentally during chewing (Fig. 1.8). When teeth are lost and are not replaced artificially the adjacent teeth may tilt and drift.

Occlusal relationships

The manner in which the opposing arches of teeth occlude is very important for function and for the comfort of the patient. It needs to be considered carefully when restoring the occluding surfaces of the teeth. The occlusion is said to be functional when:

- there is freedom for the mandible to close into maximum intercuspation in centric occlusion and centric relation,
- occlusal interfaces are free from interferences to smooth lateral and protrusive movements of the mandible, and
- occlusal contacts aid the stability of the occlusion.

The term *centric stop* refers to the occlusal contacts between supporting cusps and opposing fossae or marginal ridges in centric occlusion, that is in the position of maximum intercuspation. In the majority of dentitions the buccal cusps of the lower posterior teeth and the palatal cusps of the upper posterior teeth are supporting cusps or centric stops. Figure 1.9 demonstrates how they occlude with the opposing fossae and marginal ridges. If the centric stops are not reconstructed in a restoration, function will be reduced and uncontrolled tooth movement may result. If they are overcontoured, function will be affected, pain or discomfort may be experienced in the teeth or temporomandibular joint, and the teeth may become mobile or the restoration fracture.

In the average dentition, during protrusive movement of the mandible, the lingual surfaces of the upper anterior teeth provide anterior guidance to the opposing lower teeth. In considering lateral movements, the side to which the mandible moves at any particular time is called the working side and the other the non-working side. On the working side the buccal cusps of the lower posterior teeth may be observed to slide along the opposing cusp slopes towards or on to the buccal cusps of the upper teeth (Fig. 1.10), although in actual chewing the direction of movement

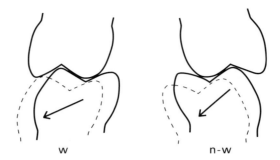

Fig. 1.10 A cross-section of molar teeth in centric occlusion seen from behind. Note the centric stops. The dotted outlines show the position which the lower teeth reach in left lateral movement on the working side (*w*) and the non-working side (*n-w*). In group function the working side buccal cusps of the lower teeth glide along the inside slopes of the buccal cusps of the upper teeth. On the non-working side the lower teeth move out of contact with the uppers.

w   n-w

is from lateral to centric. In many dentitions the canine teeth only may remain in contact. On the non-working side there should preferably be no contact between the posterior teeth due to the downward movement of the mandibular condyle on that side as it moves forward.

In abnormal conditions, with either natural or poorly restored teeth, there may be a premature contact in centric occlusion, a protrusive interference, a working side interference, or a non-working side interference. All of these are undesirable and should be corrected or, in the case of restorations, avoided.

Saliva

As well as being essential for the well-being of the mucous membranes and for swallowing, saliva bathes the teeth and helps to prevent caries. In xerostomia, the reduced secretion of saliva predisposes to the rapid development of caries.

Further reading

ASH M.M. & RAMFJORD S.P. (1982) *An Introduction to Functional Occlusion*. W.B. Saunders, Philadelphia.

SILVERSTONE L.M., JOHNSTON N.W., HARDIE J.M. & WILLIAMS R.A.D. (1981) *Dental Caries*, Part I. Macmillan, London.

Chapter 2
Prevention and treatment of dental caries

In the early days of the practice of dentistry caries was treated by extraction of the affected tooth. Later, conservation of the teeth by the removal of caries and its replacement with a filling material was practised. Today the accent is on prevention but, because complete prevention of caries presents difficulties, conservation and indeed extraction must still be practised. Nevertheless, it is still more satisfactory to prevent caries than treat it after it has already occurred. Equally, it is irrational to treat carious lesions without taking such action as is possible to prevent the recurrence of caries around the treated lesion and elsewhere in the dentition. These objectives are easy to state but difficult to achieve. The measures likely to prevent the occurrence or recurrence of caries may be considered under three headings:

- Control of the diet
- Control of the oral flora
- Control or modification of the surface layer of the tooth

Control of the diet

Dietary control consists in limiting the frequency of intake of carbohydrates, particularly monosaccharides and disaccharides. In order to educate a patient in diet control the dentist must first communicate with and then motivate his patient, and the parents if the patient is a child. He must avoid using scientific terms such as 'fermentable carbohydrates' and instead speak simply and specifically of sweets or chocolate or biscuits. Many patients, advised not to eat sweets and chocolate, may eat other types of confectionery not realising that these fall into the same category. The most satisfactory way of making this point is to ask the patient to fill in a diet sheet (Fig.2.1) listing everything he eats and drinks each day for at least three days and then analysing this with him. Positive rather than negative attitudes are the basis of all successful dietary counselling. If the emphasis is on complete prohibition, the majority of people, adult and child alike, will find

Fig. 2.1 Specimen diet record completed for 1 day.

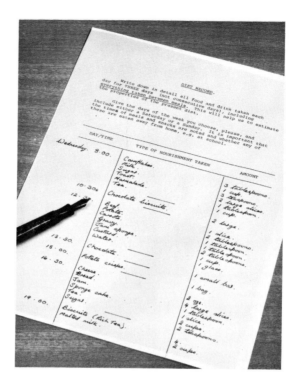

it difficult to accept the advice offered. If, however, a realistic attitude is taken, for example, that the consumption of carbohydrate is permissible at mealtimes but only at mealtimes and only if associated with oral hygiene procedures, then more patients will be likely to cooperate. The student must not only inform but also motivate. One discussion is not enough; the patient must be questioned on each visit and praised if he cooperates.

Control of the oral flora

As yet, it has proved impossible to modify the human oral flora by the use of antibiotics, vaccines or chemical agents without some risk to the patients. The long-term use of antibiotics in an attempt to control caries raises questions of bacteria becoming resistant to, or the patient becoming allergic to, the particular antibiotic used. Vaccination is still not available clinically but much progress has been made, under experimental conditions, using vaccines more sophisticated than the live ones used by Bowen (1969). The routine use of chlorhexidine mouth washes (Löe & Schiott 1970) has been limited by the associated staining of the teeth. The use of enzymes such as dextranase has not progressed since it was shown that the regular ingestion of certain of these compounds leads to a significant fall in the white cell count of monkeys (Bowen 1971).

At present the control of the oral flora must be confined to the removal of dental plaque by the traditional techniques of thorough mechanical cleansing. Efficient tooth brushing and the use of dental floss will remove plaque, including vast numbers of bacteria and their associated by-products, from the surface of the teeth. This will be particularly effective if carried out soon after meals as, by removing any recently deposited extracellular polysaccharides, it will reduce the amount of substrate available for those bacteria which remain. It has been suggested that brushing the teeth after a meal can lead to loss of surface enamel already softened by dietary and plaque acids. The alternative proposed is to remove the acidogenic plaque before the meal and before its pH can drop, but there is no long-term clinical evidence to support this technique.

Control or modification of the tooth surface

SYSTEMIC METHODS

These consist of the supplementation of the diet or drinking fluid with fluoride and possibly other trace elements. This is intended to ensure that the surface of the newly formed tooth contains the optimum amount of these constituents. The arguments for and against water fluoridation, fluoride tablets, fluoridated salt and fluoridated milk have been amply covered elsewhere (Adler 1970). Fluoridation of the water supply at a concentration of one part per million has produced decreases in caries incidence ranging between 40 and 60 per cent whilst none of the alternatives have so far produced such favourable results. Backer Dirks, Houwink & Kwant (1961) examined the effect of water fluoridation on the different surfaces of the teeth and noted a much greater caries-protective effect on the smooth surfaces of teeth than in the fissures.

LOCAL METHODS

The methods of local alteration of the tooth surface are topical fluoride applications, where the aim is to incorporate fluoride ions into the surface layer of the tooth, and the provision of a protective film on the tooth surface. The latter can be further divided into temporary films such as are produced by detergent dentifrices and more permanent films such as the fissure sealants.

Topical applications Many different techniques have been described for the application of fluoride solutions and gels to the dentition.

However, the essential features are that a medium containing free fluoride ions is brought into contact with a clean dry tooth surface in order that ionic exchange with the enamel can take place, for example, changing hydroxyapatite to fluorapatite. Szwejda (1971) reviews a variety of techniques and quotes figures of up to a 40 per cent fall in caries incidence on the smooth surfaces of the teeth. Topical application of fluoride by patients has usually consisted of the use of fluoride-containing dentifrices. This has a definite but limited caries-preventive effect. Two interesting alternatives are the mouth-rinsing techniques of Torell & Ericsson (1965) and the fluoride gel applicators of Englander *et al.* (1967), but neither of these techniques has yet achieved wide use.

Fissure sealants

The idea of treating the occlusal fissures before caries commences is attractive but not new. Hyatt (1936) advocated 'prophylactic odontomy', that is the preparation of a minimal cavity in enamel to include all the major fissures and filling it with amalgam. Fissure sealants are now available which will bond to a clean dry enamel surface that has been pretreated with acid. High retention rates and reduced caries incidence have been reported when a careful technique was used (Rock 1974).

Remineralisation As complete prevention is not always possible, the idea of reversal of the process of demineralisation in the early carious lesion should be considered. It has been possible to demonstrate the clinical remineralisation of very early carious lesions, produced experimentally in carefully chosen subjects, by improvement of the oral hygiene and the application of a fluoride solution (Fehr, Löe & Theilade 1970). The nearest approach to this phenomenon under natural conditions is the 'arresting' of an early carious lesion where for some reason, such as the extraction of the adjacent tooth or improved oral hygiene, the conditions controlling plaque formation are significantly altered.

Restoration As the progress of caries can be clinically reversed only in the early stages, it follows that the most common line of treatment once caries has occurred must be the removal of the affected tooth tissue. This can be radical, by the removal of the entire tooth, or conservative by the careful removal of the diseased tissue and its replacement by a suitable restorative material. A large part of this book is concerned with describing the planning, organisation and execution of this aspect of the conservation of teeth. Prevention must, however, never be forgotten and it will be noted how restorations are designed in combination with the more successful preventive techniques to avoid the recurrence of caries around them. Care is taken at all stages to prevent the procedures used in restoring the teeth from leading to further dental disease.

Practical preventive techniques

DIET CONTROL

An analysis of a patient's dietary habits using a diet sheet is only of value if carried out thoroughly. It must be made absolutely clear to the patient and the parent that all intake both solid and liquid must be recorded. The recording should be carried out over at least three days, one of which should be a normal school or working day and one should be at a week-end. When the records are returned it is essential to study them carefully with the patient and point out how frequently refined carbohydrate is consumed in the form of food or drink. Rational suggestions can then be made for modification of the quantity, frequency and type of food consumed.

Experiments in rodents have shown that sucrose is more cariogenic than the starches, even when the latter are cooked (Green & Hartles 1967a, b) and that the other simple sugars are also highly cariogenic (Green & Hartles 1969). Results from studies of the pH of plaque following rinsing with sucrose and glucose solutions in humans (Graf & Graf 1971) strongly suggest that the same applies in man. It has also been shown, in rats, that the inclusion of relatively small amounts of sugar in a diet either as a separate ingredient or as part of a biscuit or other confection dramatically increases its cariogenicity (Green & Hartles 1966, 1970; Ishii, König & Mühlemann 1968).

The development of caries is associated with a low plaque pH and with those sugar-containing foods which tend to keep the plaque pH low by remaining in the mouth for a long time. These foods provide readily metabolisable material for the bacteria and may be assumed to be more damaging to the teeth than those which are quickly eliminated. It would seem likely, therefore, that a sweetened drink consumed rapidly is less harmful than a slowly dissolving sweet. It has also been shown in humans (Gustafson *et al.* 1954) and in animals (König, Schmid & Schmid 1968) that increased frequency of consumption of sugars is closely correlated with an increased incidence of caries. Bearing these three factors in mind it is possible to construct two types of dietary regimen, one for the average patient, which may be regarded as a 'care and maintenance' type of regimen, and the other for patients who show a large number of active carious lesions whose control requires more stringent dietary restriction.

Standard regimen

Breakfast may well consist of cereal with possibly a little sugar or dried fruit and, if desired, a main course of bacon, eggs, sausage or possibly even cheese. Bread or toast and butter may be freely consumed preferably without jam or marmalade. Tea, coffee or milk may be taken as a beverage. Such a meal should be immediately followed by thorough oral hygiene measures.

A conventional midday meal may be taken by the average patient, although such items as toffees, biscuits or cakes with icing should be avoided. Ideally, some form of tooth cleansing should follow this meal.

A conventional evening meal may be taken and if the patient feels a compulsive need to consume biscuits, sweets or heavily iced cakes this would be the appropriate time to do so. Scrupulous oral hygiene measures should, however, be undertaken after this meal and no further food or drink should be consumed before bedtime unless it is followed by a repetition of the oral hygiene measures.

Between-meal snacks should be avoided, but if a patient considers that they are essential, milk, tea or coffee without sugar, fruit and nuts, potato crisps, bread and butter, cream crackers, totally unsweetened biscuits, and possibly ice-cream, are probably the least harmful.

Regimen for severe active caries

Breakfast may consist of cereal and milk, but this must be entirely without sugar. A main course of bacon, eggs, sausage or cheese would be acceptable and could be eaten with bread or toast and butter. No jam or marmalade may, however, be eaten with the bread or toast. Tea, coffee and milk are all acceptable drinks but once again must not be sweetened with sugar or glucose. The meal must immediately be followed by thorough oral hygiene measures.

A conventional midday meal of a cooked main course or salad may be taken. Sandwiches may be substituted but these should have a protein filling and must not contain jam, honey or any other sweetened substance. The main course may be followed by fruit or plain bread and butter. Tea, coffee or milk without sugar would be acceptable drinks. Once again, oral hygiene measures must follow this meal.

For the evening meal, a conventional main course using one of the alternatives outlined above would be acceptable followed by fruit, plain bread and butter or plain cake without filling or icing. Tea, coffee or milk without sugar would be acceptable beverages. And the meal must once again be followed by immediate oral hygiene measures.

In this regimen, no sweets, chocolate, ice-cream, fancy cake, biscuits or conserves of any kind are admissible. Between-meal snacks must be avoided completely during periods of high caries activity, but in cases of severe distress, apples, bread and butter or potato crisps could be provided.

TOPICAL APPLICATION

A simple well-proven technique for the application of fluoride solutions by the dental practitioner which is capable of convenient modification is that described by Knutson (1948). In this technique a 2 per cent solution of sodium fluoride is applied to the teeth for approximately 3 minutes. The first step is to clean the coronal surfaces of the teeth thoroughly using a rubber cup and a fine pumice paste. All traces of the paste are removed from the mouth by water spray and mouth rinsing. The cleaned teeth are then isolated using cotton wool rolls. Half the teeth present in the mouth may be treated at one time by isolating upper and lower quadrants on one side. Care must be taken to position the cotton wool rolls so that they do not absorb the applied solution. After the teeth have been isolated they are carefully dried with compressed air, particular care being given to the approximal surfaces. The fluoride solution is then applied to the dried enamel surfaces of the teeth using a small cotton applicator. If the solution is correctly applied it can be seen to wet all surfaces including the approximal ones. The solution is allowed to dry in air for approximately 3 minutes. At the end of this time, the cotton wool rolls are removed and the patient may rinse if so desired. To obtain a satisfactory caries-protective effect this procedure should be repeated on four occasions at weekly intervals. On the second, third and fourth occasions the prior prophylaxis may be omitted.

A suitable technique for the application of sodium fluoride gels under supervision either at home or in school is described by Englander *et al.* (1967). In this technique, a polyvinyl mouth piece, similar in form to an athletic mouth-guard, is made for each arch of teeth. At some convenient time each day these applicators are filled with a 1 per cent sodium fluoride gel and inserted into the mouth for 6 minutes. No attempt is made to dry the mouth or, of necessity, provide prior cleaning of the teeth with dentifrice. The use of this technique daily in a trial over a two-year period led to a noticeable reduction in the caries increment.

FISSURE SEALANTS

Although the details regarding the use of these materials vary from type to type, the more successful varieties appear to have certain features in common. After a thorough initial prophylaxis the teeth to be treated are isolated and thoroughly dried. The fissures are conditioned or lightly etched by the application of a phosphoric acid solution. After again washing and drying the surfaces, the sealant is painted over the etched areas using a fine brush or dropper. With one system the material is polymerised by the use of an intense beam of light; with others chemical activation is used.

ORAL HYGIENE

The object of oral hygiene is plaque control, that is to reduce the amount of dental plaque in the mouth to an acceptable minimum and to maintain it at this level. The patient's co-operation is essential if this is to be achieved and where this is in doubt the first stage is to demonstrate to him the presence of plaque on his teeth. This can be done by the use of disclosing tablets. These contain a red dye, erythrosin, which is released over a period of one or two minutes as they dissolve in the mouth. The dye stains the plaque which can then be readily demonstrated to the patient by means of a hand mirror and a good light.

In order to make an objective assessment of the plaque-control programme the initial level of plaque should be measured by means of a suitable index. The Debris Index component of the Oral Hygiene Index (Greene & Vermillion 1960) is particularly useful. After the patient has sucked a dissolving tablet each buccal and lingual tooth surface is scored. Where no stains or soft deposits are present a zero score is given. If soft deposits cover less than one-third of the surface or where there is extrinsic staining on any of the surface a score of 1 is recorded; for soft deposits covering between one- and two-thirds score 2, and for more than two-thirds score 3.

A plaque score for the whole mouth can be calculated but,

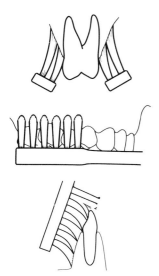

Fig. 2.2 Tooth brushing techniques. (*Upper*) angle of bristles to long axis of tooth at start of brush strokes in the buccal segments; (*centre*) correct orientation of tooth brush to occlusal plane in buccal segments; (*lower*) correct orientation of tooth brush for reaching lingual aspect of lower incisors.

except in the most extreme cases, it is the individual surface score which will be of greatest use in improving a patient's oral hygiene pattern. The teeth are carefully scaled, if necessary, and then polished. This is followed by careful instruction in appropriate oral hygiene techniques. At the next visit the Debris Index is again determined and compared with the first, both overall and surface by surface. In this way both the dentist and the patient can assess progress.

The scoring of plaque, scaling, polishing and oral hygiene instruction should be done by a dental hygienist, when one is available, but it is important that the dentist should check progress at each visit so that the patient can appreciate that the dentist feels that this aspect of treatment is important.

It is unwise to undertake advanced conservation treatment unless the Debris Index can be maintained at a suitably low level. In fact, where the dentist has a larger number of patients than he can cope with, requiring more advanced treatment, the Debris Index provides a useful method of selecting those who should receive priority. The care of patients who prove unwilling to practise effective plaque control should be restricted to the simpler forms of treatment. In explaining to the patient the value of plaque control the impression should not be given that this will effectively prevent all dental caries. Brushing techniques can effectively remove plaque from buccal and lingual surfaces and prevent smooth surface caries in these regions. This will, of course, promote gingival health but little reduction in occlusal or approximal caries has been demonstrated.

Much has been written about the necessity for adequate tooth brushing as part of oral hygiene procedures and many different methods have been described. It is, however, the thoroughness of application rather than the details of the method which is the most important factor in determining a successful result. However well a patient may appear to be following a particular method the regular use of a disclosing agent is the only reliable test of their oral hygiene. It is useful to teach one particular technique around which the patient can structure his own method. The modified Stillman method as described by Glickman (1964) provides adequate oral hygiene and is relatively easily understood by patients. The brush is positioned near the junction of the attached gingivae and the alveolar mucosa. The bristles are placed obliquely to the long axis of the tooth and directed apically (Fig. 2.2). Lateral pressure is applied against the gingivae and the brush given a rotary motion with very limited movement of the tips of the bristles. A horizontal movement must be avoided. At the same time as carrying out this slight rotary motion the handle of the brush is slowly rotated around its long axis so that the bristles of the brush pass from the attached gingivae over the marginal gingivae and the buccal or lingual aspects of the teeth. This procedure is carried out in relation to the buccal and lingual surfaces starting in the maxillary molar area, for example, and proceeding systematically throughout the mouth. To reach the lingual surfaces in the mandibular anterior area the brush is positioned so that only the two or three tufts of bristles at the tip of the brush engage the gingivae. The occlusal surfaces of the molars and premolars are scrubbed with the bristles perpendicular to the occlusal plane and penetrating into the sulci and embrasures.

Where contact between the approximal surfaces of teeth is defective, food tends to lodge in the contact area. Food debris and dental plaque can be readily removed from this area by the systematic use of dental floss. A length of dental floss approximately 8 inches long is taken and wound round one finger of either hand. The floss is then gently worked up and down through the contact area removing food debris and plaque in the process. Care must be taken at all times to avoid mechanical trauma to the interdental papilla. Various other oral hygiene aids are available such as interdental stimulators and miniature brushes. These are sometimes recommended where there has been some gingival recession but they should be used circumspectly. Care must be taken to avoid injury to the interdental papilla and the adjacent teeth when using any of these techniques.

The use of water under pressure to remove gross debris is becoming more widespread and this may be from an irrigation syringe or from an apparatus producing a pulsating water jet. The use of dental floss, water jets and other oral hygiene aids is particularly valuable where there is a greater risk of debris retention around a bridge or orthodontic appliance.

PREVENTION OF TOOTH SURFACE LOSS

As well as considering the prevention of dental caries the dentist must also concern himself with the prevention or treatment of abrasion and erosion since, when uncontrolled, these may lead to extensive loss of tooth substance, or even to the loss of teeth. Complete prevention can only come from a knowledge of the tooth brushing pattern used by the patient and his dietary habits. Early recognition of the lesions should prompt the dentist to investigate further and offer advice.

The early lesion or abrasion is easy to recognise. It is associated with gingival recession and the resultant exposure of the root of the tooth. It appears as a slight notched and polished area gingival to the enamel–cementum junction which if not arrested may progress to a deep groove between the crown and the root. The cause of this groove is the abrasive effect of enthusiastic horizontal tooth-brushing techniques.

These lesions may usually be arrested by changing to a technique employing mainly vertical strokes. Unless the patient is troubled by sensitivity to heat and cold or by the appearance of the lesions no active treatment is required. If restoration is required this can be carried out using either glass ionomer cements (Chapter 8), gold inlays, or porcelain jacket crowns (Chapter 9).

The early lesion in dental erosion is more difficult to recognise. It is usually combined with abrasion and appears smooth and polished with flattening of the developmental grooves of the labial enamel of the upper incisors out of proportion to the patient's age. Palatal and occlusal surface lesions are rarely diagnosed at an early stage.

Erosion due to acid beverages can be eliminated by avoiding this group of drinks or alleviated by the use of a drinking straw. A degree of control may be achieved by limiting the amount of fruit consumed and the anterior teeth may be further protected by dividing the fruit into segments rather than biting into it directly. Industrial erosion is prevented by wearing a soft plastic overlay covering the teeth during working hours. Cases of gastric regurgitation should be referred to a consultant. Topical fluoride application may improve the resistance of the enamel to mild acid attack. Where aesthetic or functional impairment has occurred the lesion, if small, may be restored with acid-etched composite, or if larger, with a full veneer porcelain or porcelain bonded to metal crown.

Prevention in different age groups

The advice given to individual patients must depend to a considerable extent on the condition of their mouths and in particular of their teeth and gingivae. This will be influenced by their diet, their oral hygiene, past dental treatment and especially their age.

During adolescence most patients are vulnerable to dental caries and gingival disease. The majority of the permanent posterior teeth erupt in early adolescence and these should be treated as soon as possible with topical applications of fluoride and the fissures sealed. It cannot be over-emphasised that caries and gingivitis can be effectively controlled by dietary measures and good oral hygiene. These must constitute the basis of the prescription for this age group with fluoride application, fissure sealing, orthodontic treatment and occasionally gingival recontouring as supporting measures.

In patients between 20 and 30 years old caries tends to be less of a problem but periodontal disease becomes more prevalent. Prescriptions for this age group must include measures to ensure effective interdental hygiene.

From the age of 30 into old age gingival recession and periodontal disease are the main targets for preventive measures. In cases where gingival recession has occurred cervical caries may be a problem, occurring on buccal, lingual and approximal surfaces. The treatment of caries in these regions poses many problems so effective local cleansing measures must be included in the plan. These measures must be used with care; if they are traumatic they may produce further gingival recession or abrasion cavities.

References

ADLER P. (1970) *Fluorides and Human Health*, Chapter 9. World Health Organisation, Geneva.

BACKER DIRKS O., HOUWINK B. & KWANT G.W. (1961) *Arch. oral Biol.* **5,** 284–300.

BOWEN W.H. (1969) *Brit. dent. J.* **126,** 159–160.

BOWEN W.H. (1971) *Brit. dent. J.* **131,** 445–448.

ENGLANDER H.R., KEYES P.H., GESTWICKI M. & SULTZ H.A. (1967) *J. Amer. dent. Ass.* **75,** 638–644.

FEHR VON DER F.R., LÖE H. & THEILADE E. (1970) *Caries Res.* **4,** 131–148.

GLICKMAN I. (1964) *Clinical Periodontology*, 3rd edn., p. 854. W.B. Saunders, Philadelphia.

GRAF R. & GRAF H. (1971) *Helv. odont. Acta* **15,** 42–50.

GREEN R.M. & HARTLES R.L. (1966) *Brit. J. Nutr.* **20,** 317–323.

GREEN R.M. & HARTLES R.L. (1967a) *Brit. J. Nutr.* **21,** 225–230.

GREEN R.M. & HARTLES R.L. (1967b) *Brit. J. Nutr.* **21,** 921–924.

GREEN R.M. & HARTLES R.L. (1969) *Arch. oral Biol.* **14,** 235–241.

GREEN R.M. & HARTLES R.L. (1970) *Caries Res.* **4,** 188–192.

GREENE J.C. & VERMILLION J.R. (1960) *J. Amer. dent. Ass.* **61,** 172–179.

GUSTAFSON B.E., QUENSEL C-E., LANKE L.S., LUNQVIST C., GRAHNEN H., BONOW B.E. & KRASSE B. (1954) *Acta odont. Scand.* **11,** 232–388.

HYATT T.P. (1936) *Dent. Cosmos* **78,** 353–370.

ISHII T., KÖNIG K.G. & MÜHLEMANN H.R. (1968) *Helv. odont. Acta* **12,** 41–47.

KNUTSON J.W. (1948) *J. Amer. dent. Ass.* **36,** 37–39.

KÖNIG K.G., SCHMID P. & SCHMID R. (1968) *Arch. oral Biol.* **13,** 13–26.

LÖE H. & SCHIOTT C.R. (1970) *Dental Plaque*, ed. McHugh W.D., pp. 247–256. Livingstone, Edinburgh.

LUDWIG T.G. & TAYLOR W.B. (1957) *N.Z. dent J.* **53,** 63–66.

ROCK W.P. (1974) *Brit. dent. J.* **136,** 317–321.

SZWEJDA L.F. (1971) *J. pub. Hlth. Dent.* **31,** 166–176.
TORELL P. & ERICSSON Y. (1965) *Acta odont. Scand.* **23,** 287–322.
WELLOCK W.D. & BRUDEVOLD F. (1963) *Arch. oral Biol.* **8,** 179–182.

Further reading

SILVERSTONE L.M., JOHNSON N.W., HARDIE J.M. & WILLIAMS R.A. (1981) *Dental Caries*, Part 2. Macmillan, London.

Chapter 3
Planning of treatment

The planning of treatment is one of the most important and interesting aspects of dentistry and requires a considerable breadth of knowledge and experience. On account of the introduction of new techniques, new materials and new knowledge, this is a constantly changing field providing gradual improvement in the care which can be offered. Only after observing his patients over a number of years can the dentist assess comprehensively the success or failure of his treatment plans. In difficult cases he will welcome the advice of more experienced or more specialised colleagues.

The planning of treatment involves not only the decision as to what treatment to carry out but also the sequence in which the items of treatment should be undertaken, an estimate of the time-scale involved, the cost to the patient and a realistic estimate of the prognosis. Sometimes a provisional treatment plan may have to be made initially and finalised after observing the response of the patient. Occasionally the original plan may have to be altered in the light of experience. Always the plan must be directed towards the welfare of the patient and his health, and not, more narrowly, to the restoration of the teeth. It must take the long-term view and not be confined to immediate objectives.

The essential features to be considered in making a treatment plan are:

- An assessment of the patient and his interest in his oral health
- Details of the patient's present complaint
- Dental history
- Medical history
- Family and social history
- Extra-oral examination
- Intra-oral examination
- Examination of the teeth

It is necessary to have a permanent record, to which subsequent reference can be made by the dentist, giving information regarding the history, examination, treatment plan and treatment carried out. Records must be written legibly, be concise and yet give sufficient detail, and be correctly dated and signed. Negative findings should be recorded to indicate that these particular areas have been considered and not merely omitted. Details of any accidental injury to the patient must be recorded very carefully since this may be important for medico-legal purposes. This applies whether the injury occurs during treatment or is sustained elsewhere such as in a motor vehicle accident.

ASSESSMENT OF THE PATIENT

The full name, address, telephone number, date of birth, sex, marital status, occupation and, where relevant, maiden name and code number, are recorded. In addition, a general assessment of the patient should be made noting whether he appears unwell or apprehensive, his general appearance and whether there is any difficulty in communicating with him. Further information of value in this general assessment will be obtained during the period of the history taking, examination and subsequent treatment so that the dentist will gradually improve his knowledge and understanding of the patient.

PRESENT COMPLAINT

The dentist must record the patient's complaint precisely and in sufficient detail, avoiding leading questions and if possible quoting the patient's own words. Sometimes there may be more than one complaint. If, for example, the patient feels that his denture is unsatisfactory, he should be questioned to obtain further details. Is his problem one of retention, stability, appearance, discomfort, pain or occlusal imbalance?

If the patient complains of pain then exact details must be obtained in order to improve the chance of making a correct diagnosis:

- Describe the pain in the patient's own words.
- Specify its apparent location and distribution.
- Note its character and intensity.
- Record its duration, how it began and whether it is constant or intermittent.
- Try to identify any exacerbating or relieving factors.
- Inquire about any associated symptoms.

This should be recorded in sufficient detail and include:

- The patient's previous dental treatment.
- The name and address of the dentist previously responsible for providing dental care, and the date of the last visit.
- Any difficulties experienced.
- Any previous experience of local or general anaesthesia, extractions, conservation, prosthetic or periodontal treatment.
- Details of the type of oral hygiene practised and its daily pattern.

At this stage, it may be possible for the dentist to assess the patient's attitude towards dentistry and to judge whether he has shown an active interest in maintaining his oral health or whether he is concerned only with the immediate relief of his symptoms without interest in long-term dental care.

During the interview the dentist should be alert for evidence of excessive apprehension in the patient. If he detects such evidence, he should proceed cautiously, reassuring the patient at frequent intervals.

MEDICAL HISTORY

Present

The patient should be questioned about:

- His present general health.
- The name and address of his medical practitioner.
- Whether he is currently receiving medical treatment or medication, and full details of any such medication.

Past

Detailed enquiries should be made on a systematic basis into his past medical history. The dentist should enquire about past diseases or disabilities affecting the cardiovascular system, the respiratory system and the digestive system. In particular the patient should be asked if he has, at any time, been hospitalised, suffered from rheumatic fever, valvular or other heart disease, hypertension, diabetes, epilepsy, any bleeding or clotting disorders, or any allergies. In women of childbearing age enquiries should be made to find out if the patient is pregnant. Information given by the patient should be treated as strictly confidential. If

Fig. 3.1 Instruments for intra-oral examination.
From above: mirror, pocket-measuring probe (Williams'), straight probe, Briault's probe and college tweezers.

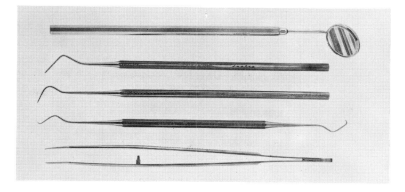

any doubt exists about the medical history or its possible effect on dental treatment the patient's medical adviser should be contacted, preferably by letter in the first instance.

FAMILY AND SOCIAL HISTORY

The patient should be asked briefly about his parents, his brothers and sisters and, depending on his age, his children. General inquiries should be made as to the pattern of dental care in his immediate family. Where hereditary abnormalities are suspected, specific enquiries should be made concerning these.

EXTRA-ORAL EXAMINATION

The extra-oral examination begins with inspection of the patient's face and neck particularly the facial contour, the lips and the maxilla–mandible relationship. Any abnormalities, such as swelling or inflammation, should be noted and investigated further. The temporomandibular joints should be palpated during opening and closing of the mouth and any abnormalities recorded. Finally the neck should be palpated for the presence of enlarged or tender lymph glands.

INTRA-ORAL EXAMINATION

For intra-oral examination the dentist requires a mirror, a straight probe, and a hooked probe such as a Briault, for checking the approximal margins of restorations. For measuring pocket depth a graduated probe such as a Williams' is required (Fig. 3.1).

The examination begins with an assessment of the appearance of the teeth and lips and the extent to which the teeth are visible during smiling and functional movements. Many patients value highly the appearance of their teeth and mouth; dentists sometimes fail to give sufficient consideration to this aspect of their patient's oral health. The dentist must record any shortcomings in the patient's dental appearance and attempt to assess the degree of the patient's concern about this. Features such as discoloration of tooth substance or restorations, lack of harmony in tooth arrangement and tooth form, and the presence of plaque and gingivitis to an extent which detracts from appearance, should be considered.

Following this the mucous membranes of the vestibule, hard and soft palates, dorsum of the tongue, under-surface of the tongue and floor of the mouth are inspected for abnormalities such as swelling, inflammation, discoloration or ulceration.

The teeth should be examined in centric occlusion and in lateral and protrusive movements. A check should be made for premature contacts in centric occlusion and interferences in protrusive, working side and non-working side contracts. Articulating paper should be used to check any suspected abnormalities. In young patients the classification of any malocclusion should be noted. The extent to which loss of teeth has reduced function should be assessed.

The teeth should be percussed by tapping with the end of the mirror handle and any increased sensitivity should be recorded. The teeth should be checked individually for mobility by attempting to move them buccally and lingually using a finger and a mirror handle and the degree of mobility recorded. The presence of plaque and calculus must be noted and disclosing tablets may be used to demonstrate the presence of plaque to the patient. The gingivae should be examined for abnormalities, in particular the presence of inflammation. Where gingival disease is present a pocket measuring probe should be used and the depth of pockets in excess of 2 mm should be charted. This should not be done in patients who are at risk of bacterial endocarditis unless an antibiotic cover is being used.

Where dentures are present they should be inspected carefully for appearance, retention, stability, comfort and function. In saddle areas the condition of the mucosa and the contour of the underlying bone should be checked.

EXAMINATION AND CHARTING OF THE TEETH

The teeth must be inspected for the presence of abnormalities including caries, restorations either defective or sound and excessive tooth surface loss. The absence or partial eruption of teeth and the presence of roots should be noted. This examination

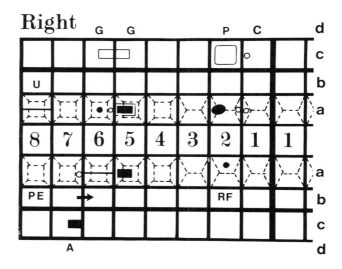

Fig. 3.2 Right half of a charting grid. The explanation is given in the text.

should be done systematically. One such system is to start with the upper right third molar and proceed via the upper anterior teeth to the upper left quadrant and from there to the lower left quadrant, lower anterior teeth and lower right quadrant. Details of the findings should be recorded on the charting grid (Fig. 3.2) using one of the established conventions.

The charting grid is designed to give a graphic representation of the patient's teeth. There are a number of designs in use; all of them indicate, by means of a diagrammatic or pictorial design, each of the 32 permanent teeth and usually the 20 deciduous teeth. On these charting grids are indicated the extent of restorations, of cavities, of restorations to be re-made, the state of tooth eruption and drifting of the teeth.

The chart in Fig. 3.2 covers the upper and lower teeth of the right side. The terms right and left always refer to the patient's right and left sides. By convention the charting is always arranged as if the dentist were viewing the patient from the front, face to face. The squares have divisions representing the mesial, distal, buccal or labial, and lingual surfaces. The molar and premolar squares contain an additional central square for the occlusal surface. The lingual surfaces are those adjacent to the numbers. Number 1 represents the central incisor, number 2 the lateral incisor and so on. The rows labelled 'a' are used to indicate the state of the teeth at examination making use of symbols. Thus caries requiring treatment is indicated by an outline extending over the surface or surfaces involved, an existing restoration by a shaded area covering the surfaces involved, a restoration to be re-made by a combination of these, namely a line enclosing a shaded area and a missing tooth by a horizontal line. It is particularly important that representations of cavities and fillings are accurately confined to the surfaces involved; the charting is symbolic, not topographical. The original charting is not altered subsequently other than to correct omissions.

The rows labelled 'b' are used for observations not recorded in row 'a'. Thus, U indicates an unerupted tooth; PE a partially erupted tooth; A an artificial tooth on a denture; RF a root-filled tooth; CR a crown; and BR a bridge. The rows labelled 'c' show the restorations which are planned. They are drawn in as open spaces at the time of planning treatment and are filled in as the restorations are completed. Thus one can easily see the progress which has been made at any time. The materials to be used in the planned restorations are indicated in rows 'd'. A indicates amalgam, C composite, G gold, P porcelain and so on.

The charting in Fig. 3.2 indicates that the upper right third molar is unerupted, the second molar is sound, the first molar has an occlusal filling and a mesial cavity and it is planned to restore this by means of a mesio-occlusal gold inlay. The second premolar has a defective disto-occlusal filling which it is planned to remake as a gold inlay. The first premolar and the canine are sound. The lateral incisor has a distal restoration involving the incisal edge and a mesial cavity and is to have a porcelain crown. The central incisor has a distal cavity to be restored. In the lower arch the third molar is partially erupted. The second molar has a mesial cavity which has been restored by means of a mesio-occlusal amalgam filling since the charting was made; the first molar is missing and the second molar has moved mesially. The second premolar has a disto-occlusal restoration, the first premolar, canine and central incisor are sound while the lateral incisor has been root filled and has a lingual restoration.

Tooth notation

A number of systems are used to designate individual teeth by means of a shorthand system. The notation currently used in Britain is indicated in Fig. 3.3. However, the system adopted by the FDI (*Fédération Dentaire Internationale*) seems likely to become more widely used (Fig. 3.4). It has the advantage of being suitable for computerisation, is more convenient for typing and printing and may reduce the risk of error. Thus the permanent lower left second molar is designated $\overline{7}$ in the present notation or 37 in the FDI system.

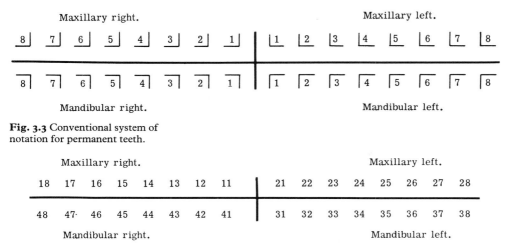

Fig. 3.3 Conventional system of notation for permanent teeth.

Fig. 3.4 FDI system for notation for permanent teeth.

Study casts

In any patient where partial dentures or bridges are being considered, or where the treatment plan is not straightforward, impressions should be taken and study casts prepared and mounted on an average path or semi-adjustable articulator. These casts are invaluable in treatment planning since they show some features difficult to see in the mouth. They enable the dentist to consider the treatment plan at leisure and to discuss it with his technician.

Further examination

Pathological examinations, such as bleeding and clotting times, haemoglobin levels or biopsies will be required in some cases.

RADIOGRAPHIC EXAMINATION

Radiographic examination of the crowns of posterior teeth is best carried out by means of bitewing radiography, using a film with a tab projecting horizontally from one side. The patient bites on the tab and this holds the film vertically on the lingual side of the teeth. The X-ray tube is positioned almost horizontally and aligned so that the beam passes between the contact areas and no overlapping of the approximal surfaces appears on the radiograph. Periapical radiographs of the lower posterior teeth also give a satisfactory

Fig. 3.5 Diagram of teeth as seen on a bitewing radiograph. The second molar tooth has an occlusal metal restoration with a cement lining; the underlying dentine shows sclerosis. The first molar has occlusal and distal caries involving the enamel and dentine. The premolar has a cervical radiolucency mesially. The pulp chambers are large as in a young patient.

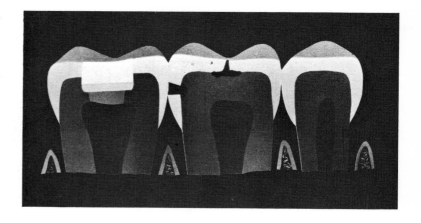

picture of their crowns but this is not the case with upper teeth, unless the long cone technique is used. Periapical views of incisor and canine teeth are satisfactory for examination of their crowns. Panoramic radiographs are valuable for giving a general scan of the teeth, maxilla and mandible.

In order to make a diagnosis the radiographs must have satisfactory contrast, projection and definition as well as being free from artifacts.

Diagnosis should not be attempted from films which are inadequate in any of these respects. A radiograph of the crown of a tooth should show the outline of the pulp chamber in section and should clearly differentiate between the enamel and the dentine (Fig. 3.5). Radiographs of some teeth show radiolucent areas mesially and distally in the region of the enamel–cementum junction (Fig. 3.6). Usually these are artifacts associated with two features, the absence of a covering layer of enamel or bone and the presence of a convexity or concavity which is less of a barrier to X-rays than a flat surface.

Restorative materials containing heavy atoms appear as radio-opaque areas which appear dense white when held in front of a light. These materials include amalgam, gold, zinc cements and others to which a radio-opaque material, such as barium salt, has been added. Composites are radiolucent and calcium hydroxide cement is only slightly radio-opaque but a more radio-dense material is sometimes added to these.

Diagnosis of approximal caries is best made from good bitewing radiographs (Fig. 3.7). These radiographs should be checked to ensure that they are correctly orientated on their mount. This is done by placing each film with the convexity of the embossed

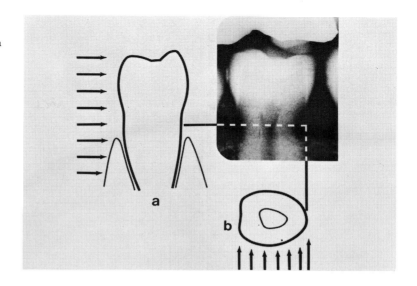

Fig. 3.6 The cervical radiolucency, frequently seen on an intra-oral radiograph, resembles a carious lesion but is usually an artifact due to the X-rays reaching this area being absorbed to a lesser extent than elsewhere, (*a*) due to the absence of enamel and bone and (*b*) to a convexity or concavity on the approximal surface of the root.

marker spot towards the observer, orienting the films so that the upper teeth are above and the lower teeth below and so that the premolars are mesial to the molars. Examination of the radiographs should proceed systematically from one side to the other checking each diagnostically important feature.

Bitewing radiographs do not show occlusal carious lesions until these have reached at least a moderate size. Approximal caries usually becomes visible some time before the lesion reaches the dentine (Fig. 3.7). Generally it has progressed substantially further clinically than appears to be the case on radiographic examination. It is difficult to judge accurately the proximity of deep caries to the pulp. Secondary dentine may be visible on the radiograph, just as is primary dentine, but the difference between the two is not usually obvious. Under some amalgam restorations a radio-opaque zone, shaped like a truncated cone, may be seen (Fig. 3.8). This has been shown to be due to tin and zinc particles passing into demineralised dentine (Kurosaki & Fusayama 1973). Pulp stones are occasionally visible on radiographs but generally have little clinical significance.

In the case of teeth having extensive caries or extensive restorations it is advisable to have periapical radiographs to aid in determining the condition of the root canal and periapical bone (Fig. 3.9). These may show the existence of a periapical rarefaction, representing a granuloma or abscess, related to teeth with

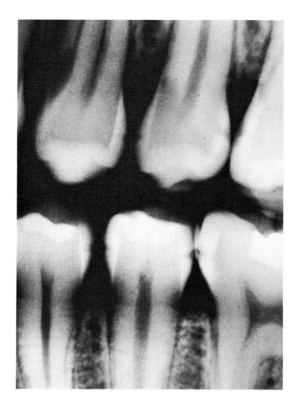

Fig. 3.7 Bitewing radiograph showing caries on almost every approximal surface. On the distal surface of the upper second premolar the dentine may be involved but on other surfaces only the enamel appears to be involved. For these surfaces the institution of preventive measures with regular radiographic controls is indicated. Note again the cervical radiolucency, particularly on the lower premolar teeth.

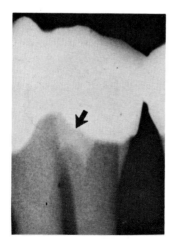

Fig. 3.8 Area of radiopacity (*arrow*) below a metal restoration.

necrotic pulps. They will show the presence of an existing root filling and are a necessary preliminary to endodontic treatment (Fig. 3.10).

Sequence and phases of treatment planning

While each treatment plan must be made on an individual basis, some general principles can be laid down as a guide to the student, particularly with regard to the sequence in which treatment should be carried out.

EMERGENCY TREATMENT

Treatment for relief of pain or discomfort should be given priority. Apart from the obvious need to make the patient comfortable, successful relief of pain may support his confidence in the dentist. Generally this consists of excavating and dressing a

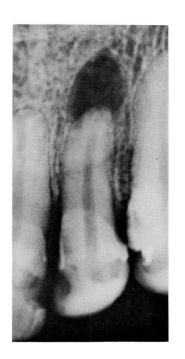

carious lesion, removal of a damaged pulp in preparation for a subsequent root filling, or extraction of a tooth.

PREVENTIVE MEASURES

The temporary treatment of advanced caries by excavation and dressing of a cavity will usually prevent pain and limit further progress of caries until a permanent restoration can be made. This will also enable the dentist to make an accurate assessment of the prognosis and the treatment planned for each tooth.

The removal of plaque and calculus and the instruction of the patient in oral hygiene should be carried out early in a course of treatment. This will allow the dentist to assess the success of the patient's oral hygiene measures and give him the opportunity to correct deficiencies before the treatment is completed. It will allow a more precise examination and will also reduce haemorrhage from inflamed gingivae thus facilitating conservative procedures.

The prevention of new carious lesions by diet control and topical measures should be instituted at this stage. In patients who are particularly susceptible to caries, reparative procedures not accompanied by caries control measures, will be of limited value.

REASSESSMENT

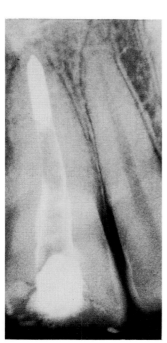

At this stage the results of the preventive measures detailed above should be reviewed and considered in conjunction with the extent and type of further treatment which has been provisionally planned. Unless a patient is able to attend as required and to co-operate effectively in oral hygiene and diet control, it is unwise to attempt extensive or complex restorative treatment. Instead, the dentist should simplify the plan and try to provide only basic treatment. This might involve, for example, the extraction of extensively carious teeth and the provision of a simple partial denture instead of root fillings and crowns. Indeed, some dentists feel that no permanent treatment should be provided until the patient achieves and maintains satisfactory plaque control.

It is worth making the point that it is never simple to influence the unmotivated patient to practise effective preventive measures. This requires frequent and repeated efforts on the part of the

Fig. 3.9 (*above*) Part of a periapical radiograph showing an apical area of radiolucency on an upper left lateral incisor.

Fig. 3.10 (*below*) Part of a periapical radiograph showing an apical third root filling in an upper left central incisor. The fractured crown has not yet been permanently restored.

dentist and the dental hygienist. In such patients it may be useful to calculate the Debris Index before oral hygiene measures are commenced, and again at intervals so that both the dentist and the patient can have an objective assessment of the effectiveness of plaque control measures.

GENERAL TREATMENT

● Where partial dentures or bridges are required the detailed design must be finalised at this stage. This will enable the correct restorations to be planned to allow for the inclusion of rest seats, parallel guiding planes, retention for clasps or the fitting of precision attachments.
● Extraction of teeth to be replaced by dentures or bridges should be carried out early to allow time for alveolar remodelling. If necessary temporary dentures should be constructed.
● Where periodontal surgery is required it is not always easy to decide whether to carry it out before, or after, restorations involving the gingival margins. If the periodontal surgery is carried out first it will simplify the restorative procedures. On the other hand, open contacts or poorly contoured temporary dressings will aggravate the periodontal condition and make hygiene difficult. Possibly the best solution is to make well-contoured semi-permanent restorations until after the periodontal surgery has been completed and the gingivae have healed.
● The restoration of individual teeth should be carried out at this stage. This is best done in quadrants so as to simplify anaesthesia and impression taking and will cause less disturbance to the patient. The restorations should be polished. Bridges may be completed as part of this phase of treatment.
● Partial dentures should be completed.

FOLLOW-UP

Arrangements should be made to recall the patient after a suitable interval which may vary from three months to six months or one year.

Diagnosis of caries

The decision as to whether or not to restore a tooth poses little problem when a definite cavity exists and the tooth is judged to be worth retaining. It is then quite clear that, if the tooth is not restored, the caries will progress and lead to the loss of the tooth.

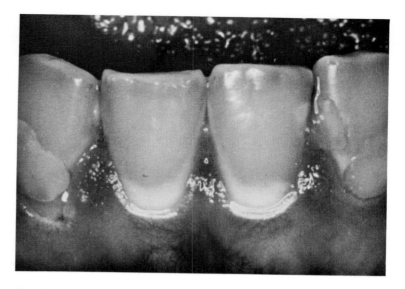

Fig. 3.11 Arrested early enamel caries at the cervical region of lower central incisors. This was treated two years previously by plaque control and topical fluoride gel applications. The enamel surface still has a white opaque appearance but is hard.

In the young patient this will happen more rapidly than in the older patient. However, at an early stage in the carious process the decision is less easy. The question to be asked and answered is: will the caries progress if the tooth is not filled in spite of any preventive measures it may be possible to adopt? Fortunately, the decision is not critical if the tooth can be kept under regular observation and there is also value in postponing the restoration and observing the effect of preventive measures.

Early cervical caries, showing a white, dull, slightly soft enamel surface without cavitation, is more amenable to preventive measures than caries in other regions. With reasonable patient co-operation it is not difficult to eliminate plaque from this region by brushing. Frequent topical applications of fluoride gel can effectively build up the resistance of the enamel surface and perhaps bring about some remineralisation (Fig. 3.11). These measures coupled with diet control can effectively prevent the extension of caries in this region and should be adopted before considering cavity preparation and restoration. Even if a small area of cavitation exists it may be wise, in co-operative patients, to restore it without extension initially and to attempt to obtain arrest of the remainder of the lesion in order to avoid an otherwise extensive restoration.

Early approximal caries is diagnosed from radiographs. Where an adjacent tooth is present it is not possible to diagnose it at an early stage by clinical examination. The carious lesion tends to be further advanced than its radiographic appearance would suggest.

If the lesion appears to have reached the dentine there is no doubt that it should be restored. If, however, the lesion does not appear to have reached the dentine the dentist should attempt to produce arrest of caries (Rugg-Gunn 1972) by means of diet control, topical fluoride applications and the use of floss interdentally. In some cases these measures will fail because the caries was more advanced than was apparent. If the patient cannot be kept under observation or if preventive measures cannot be successfully applied then it may be better to restore the tooth at an early stage.

Occlusal caries is more difficult to arrest. The traditional test for cavitation in occlusal fissures is the use of a sharp probe which is found to penetrate some distance into the fissure. Since fissure caries progresses more rapidly in young patients than in old patients, it is wise in the younger patient to cut out and restore heavily stained deep fissures where there is any sign of cavitation. In older patients, stained shallow fissures are frequently found which may not progress to cavitation and with these it may be best to delay treatment. Radiographs are of little value in the early diagnosis of occlusal caries.

DECISION TO RESTORE A TOOTH

In the previous section it was made clear that when a definite cavity exists in a tooth, which is deemed to be valuable, the tooth should be treated by cavity preparation and restoration. This statement raises the question of deciding on the value of the tooth since if a tooth is of no value there is little point in making the effort to restore it. This is particularly the case where the tooth is functionless, or unlikely to become functional, and as a result may pose difficulty in cleaning together with the risk of over-eruption. We have already stressed the importance of considering the dentition as a whole but within this context it is still necessary to consider individual teeth.

The value of a tooth may be considered under a number of headings:

● Aesthetic
● Functional, including mastication and speech
● Orthodontic
● Prosthetic

If a tooth contributes to appearance, or function or is valuable or likely to become valuable to form support for a partial denture or bridge, then it should be restored. Canine teeth and single molar teeth in good alignment are generally valuable as abutment teeth.

If there is crowding in a segment of the mouth and a need for reduction in the number of teeth, then it may be wiser to sacrifice a carious tooth rather than a sound tooth.

If the restoration of a tooth poses a difficult problem one may have to assess the value of the tooth in relation to the difficulty of restoration. For example, a valuable tooth may be worth a considerable effort in making a restoration while a tooth of marginal value may not.

Replacing a faulty restoration

Research by Elderton (1977) has demonstrated that, in practice, when a restoration is replaced, major defects in the previous restoration may be corrected but minor deficiencies will still be present around the new restoration. Clear evidence of caries or a distinct defect must, therefore, be present before it is decided to replace a restoration. Indeed, with large and particularly pin-retained restorations, consideration should be given to retaining the sound part of the restoration whilst removing and replacing the defective area.

Planning of treatment for patients with medical problems

In patients suffering from certain systemic diseases the provision of dental treatment introduces problems which, if not foreseen, may lead to serious consequences. For the most part problems arise from dental treatment of a surgical nature but in some cases special care has to be taken in the conservation of teeth.

Cardiovascular disease

In patients who have suffered from rheumatic fever, chorea or bacterial endocarditis or who are affected by congenital heart disease, valvular heart disease or who have been treated by cardiac surgery, there is a risk of precipitating an attack of sub-acute bacterial endocarditis if a bacteraemia involving certain organisms, particularly streptococcus viridans, is caused during the course of dental treatment.

In such cases it is necessary to protect the patient against this possibility by arranging for a cover of an appropriate antibiotic. While some authorities recommend this precaution for all restorations, the authors consider that it is only indicated where manipulation of the gingival tissue is involved as in the preparation and restoration of cavities which extend sub-gingivally. In such cases antibiotic cover should be given so as to produce an adequate blood level at the time the procedure is carried out.

Bleeding and clotting disorders

These include patients suffering from haemophilia, Christmas disease, purpura and patients suffering from cardiovascular disease who are receiving anticoagulant therapy. The risk of gingival haemorrhage in these patients during conservation treatment is not serious, but bleeding into the tissues following an injection of local anaesthetic solution may cause extensive bruising. In the case of an inferior dental block this may spread to the spaces of the neck and lead to difficulty in respiration.

Patients receiving medication

Patients receiving certain drugs require special care during conservation treatment. Patients on tricyclic antidepressant drugs should not be given local anaesthetic containing noradrenaline or adrenaline. The risk in giving injections of local anaesthetic to patients on anticoagulant drugs has already been mentioned. Patients receiving systemic corticosteroids are not generally affected by routine conservation treatment and so seldom need to have their dosage increased prior to treatment, but the advice of their physician should be sought.

The management of chronically ill patients

Prolonged sessions and courses of dental treatment should be avoided in patients who are chronically ill or debilitated. In patients whose life expectancy is limited, such as in chronic leukaemia, semi-permanent restorations may be indicated to alleviate oral manifestations and sustain morale.

Risk to the dentist

Some contagious or infectious diseases, such as serum hepatitis, from which patients may suffer, involve a risk to the dentist. If he is aware of the patient's condition he may either take suitable precautions (Chapter 13) or postpone elective treatment until there is less risk to himself. The dentist must also be aware of the possibility of an infectious or contagious disease being transferred to a subsequent patient.

The elderly patient

Dental care of elderly people is subject to a variety of constraints. They may be chronically unwell, unable to travel to the surgery or may find it difficult to tolerate long sessions of treatment. They adapt poorly to the loss of teeth and the disturbance of neuro-muscular mechanisms consequent on this and on the fitting of dentures. With the relatively short life expectancy of the patient, preservation of a tooth for three or four years may be very important. In the elderly, inability to provide an 'ideal' restoration is not justification for extraction. Compromise and understanding are the keys to treatment.

The advent of self-threading pins and adhesive restorative materials have made the short-term restoration of their dentitions simpler. The highest level of skill must be applied but it is the actual service to the patient which is the overriding concern.

Low-seated dentistry

The treatment of patients in a horizontal position probably reduces the risk of a vaso-vagal attack, but a substantial number of patients dislike, at least initially, being treated in this position. It may pose difficulties in respiration for patients who do not have a clear nasal airway and be unpleasant for those with a hiatus hernia.

Patients in special need of routine dental care

While routine dental care is desirable for all patients who require it there are some in whom its absence may lead to serious difficulties. Patients suffering from physical handicaps involving their hands may find their teeth invaluable for some activities for which hands are normally used. The loss of teeth may lead to a serious increase in their handicap and so careful conservation treatment is required. In patients who have received radiation therapy to the dental areas of the mandible and maxilla there may be a risk of radionecrosis if extractions have to be carried out. It follows therefore that every effort should be made to maintain the teeth in a healthy condition to avoid this risk. Patients in whom teeth are used for accessory functions, such as playing a wind instrument, require exceptional care to avoid loss of teeth, particularly anterior teeth. Palatal defects following surgery or congenital abnormalities may lead to problems in the construction of full or even partial dentures and special efforts should be directed towards the maintenance of the dentition.

Treatment planning for patients with extensive caries

Not infrequently the dentist is faced with the problem of planning treatment for a patient suffering from extensive dental caries. Many of these patients are children in their early teens whose teeth do not have a high resistance to caries and have been exposed to a highly cariogenic environment. They may not have received dental treatment, either because of apprehension or through lack of interest on the part of their parents. Another group of patients which poses similar problems includes adults who have numerous extensive restorations which are defective. This condition may arise through the neglect on the part of the patient to practise effective oral hygiene and diet control and to obtain regular dental treatment, or it may arise through a dentist neglecting to provide adequate dental care. In any event this poses a considerable problem to the dentist, first in planning treatment, and second in carrying it out.

HISTORY AND EXAMINATION

A complete history and examination should be carried out along the lines described earlier, but certain points are worthy of special consideration. During the history the patient's attitude to dental care and oral hygiene should be assessed and an attempt made to ascertain why adequate treatment was not carried out at an earlier stage. Details of any symptoms are important since they may indicate the need for emergency treatment and may contribute to the diagnosis of pulp disease.

It is important to obtain a pan-oral radiograph, or periapical views if necessary, to show the condition of the periapical regions and to obtain bitewing radiographs to indicate the presence and extent of carious lesions, particularly approximal caries. A dietary investigation is essential. At the same time the dentist should ascertain whether the patient has any difficulty in attending for a course of treatment.

TREATMENT PLANNING

Some of the difficulty experienced by students in planning treatment for patients with extensive caries arises from the feeling that a definitive treatment plan should be reached on the first or second visit. This is generally not advisable; instead, the student should conceive of treatment being carried out in three phases:

● A preliminary period of assessment

- A period of repair
- A period of control

Period of assessment

The dentist should at an early stage arrive at a preliminary treatment plan. As part of this plan he should carry out certain procedures:

- Assessment of each carious tooth with regard to the difficulty of restoration.
- Control of existing caries by the use of temporary restorations to prevent its further spread.
- Prevention of further caries by oral hygiene, topical fluoride application and fissure sealants.

The dentist should also motivate his patient as far as possible to carry out a regimen designed to reduce to a minimum the occurrence of new carious lesions. This will include effective oral hygiene, diet control and the need for regular attendance. Advice regarding diet control must be radical since, unless caries control is completely effective, the prognosis is very poor indeed.

During the preliminary period of assessment the dentist will be able to determine the reaction of the patient to treatment and his response in terms of satisfactory oral hygiene and diet control.

Period of repair

At the end of the preliminary period of assessment the dentist must arrive at a definitive treatment plan. Prior to this he may need to carry out a new examination for caries since, initially, the presence of debris may have prevented a thorough examination. In general, three main lines of treatment are possible:

- *Conservation of all or almost all teeth* This line of treatment may require a considerable amount of work and priority should be given to those patients in whom effective co-operation has been obtained. Where the patient is apprehensive, or travels a long distance, consideration should be given to the use of sedation or general anaesthesia in order to carry out the maximum amount of treatment in one visit. Where possible, full coverage restorations such as crowns are advantageous since they reduce the risk of further caries. Treatment should be carried out in quadrants, but when replacing a number of extensive restorations it is wise to treat only one quadrant at a time.

● *Conservation of some teeth,* the extraction of others and the provision of partial dentures. The dentures should be designed to have minimum contact with the teeth so as to reduce the risk of plaque retention and caries. Preference should be given to retaining those teeth of greatest prosthetic value; in the upper arch, the canine and second molar teeth are often of most importance while in the lower arch the incisor, canine and premolar teeth may often be retained and where possible a molar tooth on each side should be preserved to assist the stability of the denture.

● *Clearance of one or both arches* This may be carried out at once or may be delayed. The provision of immediate dentures is desirable.

Period of control

Where any teeth have been retained it is very important to institute a regular follow-up at six-monthly intervals, or more frequently if considered advisable, so that reinforcement of oral hygiene and diet control can be carried out. Particularly in older patients, where full coverage restorations have been extensively used and caries control has been effective, the frequency with which further restorations are required should decline markedly.

References

ELDERTON R.J. (1977) *Assessment of the Quality of Dental Care.* Ed. H. Allred. pp. 45–81. London Hospital Medical College.

KUROSAKI N. & FUSAYAMA T. (1973) *J. dent. Res.* **52,** 309–316.

RUGG-GUNN A.J. (1972) *Brit. dent. J.* **133,** 481–484.

Chapter 4
Instruments and minor equipment

The preparation of hard dental tissues to receive a filling or restoration is carried out by means of rotary cutting and grinding tools and hand instruments. Rotary instruments are also used in the shaping, finishing and polishing of restorations both in the mouth and in the laboratory. Hand instruments are required for inserting cements and filling materials, for carving wax and amalgam, and in the examination of the mouth. Both hand instruments and vibrating instruments are effective in condensing amalgam.

Until the early part of the nineteenth century tooth preparation was carried out exclusively with hand instruments. They were heavy, cumbersome and made of inferior metal by the standards of today. Some were operated by hand pressure or by the use of a small mallet and some, in the shape of a bur, were rotated by hand. These early hand instruments later became standardised into the patterns which we know today.

During the nineteenth century hand-operated mechanical systems such as drills operated by bow strings, by Archimedian drives, and by rack and pinion drives came into use. A considerable advance was made in the late nineteenth century with the introduction of a pedal-driven engine connected by a flexible cable drive to a handpiece into which could be fitted individual burs. This gave higher speeds, simpler and more positive control of the handpiece and permitted a range of shapes and sizes of burs to be used. The first power drill was operated by a clockwork motor and towards the end of the nineteenth century electric motors began to be employed, but it was many years before they superseded the foot engine. The flexible cable was replaced by a cord arm drive, or endless cord running over a system of pulleys; this was more efficient and allowed greater speeds than the cable drive but was still rather awkward to use. Up to 1940 few dentists were using bur speeds greater than 5000 r.p.m. In the 1950s systems of gears, fitted either externally at the end of the handpiece or internally, were introduced which, together with a larger driving pulley on the electric motor, increased speeds to 40 000 r.p.m.

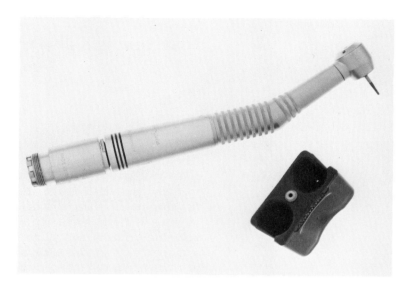

In 1957 the Borden Airotor, an air-driven turbine handpiece, came on the market and it quickly became obvious that this was the instrument for which dentists had been waiting. Driven by compressed air carried through a flexible tube and with a small turbine mounted on two ball races in the head of a contra-angle handpiece, it produced speeds of about 300,000 r.p.m. when running free but less than this under load. Not long afterwards the air-bearing turbine handpiece, with air-bearings in place of ball-bearings, was introduced (Fig. 4.1). It gave free-running speeds of up to 500,000 r.p.m. and a reduction in noise level compared to the earlier turbines.

On account of the absence of a direct drive, turbine handpieces produce a lower torque or twisting force than conventional handpieces. In clinical terms this means that if the operator presses too hard on the handpiece during cutting the bur will stall, and so he must learn to use the correct pressure to produce the highest possible rate of cutting. The high rate of cutting and the absence of any tendency for burs to skid allow more delicate and precise handling with less fatigue of the operator's fingers. The Borden type has been largely superseded by higher torque turbines, with either air bearings or ball races (Fig. 4.1). These have larger heads to accommodate the larger turbines but are shaped to improve visibility.

The air motor and the electric micro-motor were introduced for operations requiring lower speeds and greater torque (Fig. 4.2). The air-motor is an air-driven motor fitted at the end of the

Fig. 4.2 Air motor (*above*): contra-angle handpiece accepting latch type burs (*centre*); straight handpiece accepting latch type burs (*bottom*). The tube carrying air and water is connected to the left side of the air motor; the handpieces fit on to the drive shaft on the right. The two holes, separated off by O rings, allow air and water separately to reach the head of the handpiece to provide a cooling spray.

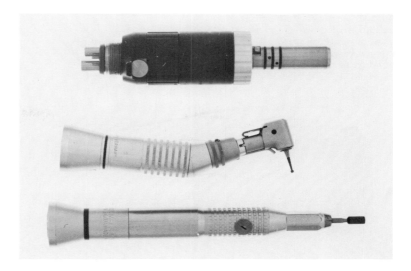

handpiece, while the micro-electric motor is a miniaturised electric motor fitted at the same point. When used with speed-increasing and speed-reducing geared handpieces these motors can operate in a range from about 600 r.p.m. to 120,000 r.p.m. with adequate torque and a low noise level. The air-motor is simpler because it needs no electrical supply and it is replacing the micro-motor.

Early dental handpieces were of two kinds; the straight handpiece which held the bur in a compression grip and the right-angle handpiece which used a latch to hold the bur in position. The right-angle handpiece was superseded by the contra-angle handpiece which, by bringing the head of the bur into line with the axis of the handpiece shaft, gave greater control since the handpiece did not tend to turn in the operator's hand. The air turbine handpiece has a contra-angle shape and makes use of a tightly fitting sleeve to retain the bur, which is therefore known as a friction grip bur. Higher bur speeds brought with them the problem of pulp damage due to the heat produced during cutting. This problem was largely solved by incorporating into the handpiece an air and water spray directed at the cutting part of the bur.

Rotary instruments

DESIGN OF BURS

A typical bur consists of three parts, the shank, the neck and the head.

Fig. 4.3 Burs designed for different handpieces.
(*Top*) for straight handpiece with compression grip; (*centre left*) latch-type bur; (*centre right*) latch-type bur for miniature handpiece; (*bottom*) friction grip bur.

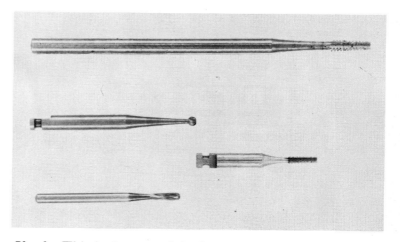

Shank This is the part of the instrument which is held in the handpiece and is shaped according to the method of its retention (Fig. 4.3). The shank for the traditional straight handpiece is cylindrical and is retained in the handpiece by a compression grip. The shank for the angle handpiece is shorter, has a groove near its end which is used to retain it in the handpiece by means of a latch, and a flat surface at the end so that the rotary force can be applied without slip occurring. It is called a latch type bur. A similar but shorter type of shank is used in the miniature handpiece designed for use in children or where access is restricted. More recently, straight handpieces have been designed to make use of latch type burs and so reduce the range of burs which the dentist must keep. The friction grip shank is shorter and thinner and is designed for the air turbine and some other high-speed handpieces. It is held in position by being pressed into a tightly fitting chuck. A special tool is provided for inserting and removing the bur; failure to use this may lead to bending of the bur or damage to the bearings of the handpiece (Fig. 4.1). In some modern turbine handpieces the insertion and removal of the bur is controlled by a press button on the head of the handpiece.

Neck Except for larger instruments, the neck normally tapers from the shank to a smaller diameter related to the size of the head of the bur. This taper improves visibility and allows greater freedom of manipulation within a cavity.

Head The cutting and grinding heads of dental burs are manufactured in a variety of materials (Fig. 4.4). Steel burs are used for cutting dentine but are inefficient for cutting enamel and

Fig. 4.4 Burs of different types. *From left:* steel cross-cut fissure bur, tungsten carbide plain-cut fissure bur, tapered fissure finishing bur, diamond fissure bur, silicon carbide stone.

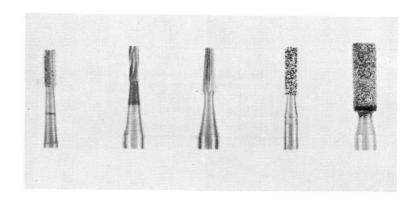

suitable for low speeds only. They are, however, relatively cheap. Tungsten carbide burs have heads of tungsten carbide welded to a steel shank and neck. This material is much harder than steel and is effective for cutting enamel and producing precise shapes in tooth preparation. These burs may fracture if used carelessly. Steel and tungsten carbide burs have blades and are classed as cutting instruments. On the other hand, a variety of rotary instruments consisting of an abrasive material bonded on to a metal core, are classed as grinding instruments. The commonest of these are diamond burs and silicon carbide stones. Diamond burs are effective in cutting enamel and amalgam but do not give the precision of shape or smoothness of cavity finish produced by cutting instruments.

Shape Different shapes of dental cutting instruments are available; the most useful are shown in Fig. 4.5. Grinding instruments are made in an even greater variety of shapes.

Size Cutting and grinding instruments are manufactured in various sizes. Many steel burs are available in twelve or fourteen sizes and tungsten carbide burs in four or five. An individual dentist does not need the complete range that is available and should rationalise his bur selection to a relatively small number.

Cutting instruments These are manufactured with a number of different designs of blades. Most burs have blades which are set at a slight angle so that they spiral round the bur and give a more even cutting and planing action. Some, known as plain-cut burs, have continuous blades. Others, known as cross-cut burs, have blades which are notched at intervals. They were originally designed before high speeds became available to improve the rate of cutting

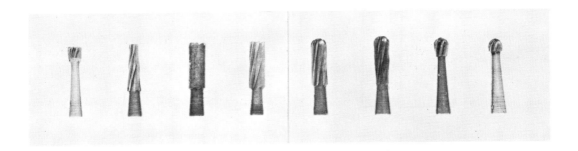

Fig. 4.5 Burs of different shapes. *From left:* inverted cone, plain-cut tapered fissure, end-cutting, plain-cut fissure; dome-ended fissure, long pear, short pear, round.

enamel but it is doubtful if they have much value now. The cutting edges are set at an angle so that they cut only while rotating in a clockwise direction. Other steel burs, known as finishing burs, have finer and more numerous blades which have a straight, not spiral, pattern. They are used for finishing the margins of cavities and the surfaces of restorations before polishing. Tungsten carbide blanks, known as Baker-Curson burs, are used for final finishing.

Grinding instruments

These consist of small angular particles of a very hard abrasive substance bonded to a core of metal. Parts of the abrasive particles project beyond the surface of the bonding material and it is these which produce the grinding action. If the particles are large and project far beyond the surface they provide rapid cutting and a rough surface finish; small particles which project only slightly produce slower cutting and a smoother surface.

Finishing and polishing equipment

Polishing is the production of a smooth shiny surface on a material as the result of the formation of an amorphous surface layer. It is achieved by grinding the surface with successively finer abrasives and polishing agents until a mirror-like finish is produced. The fine abrasives can be applied in the form of rotating discs coated with abrasive particles, or soft cups and discs incorporating the particles, which wear away rapidly exposing a new abrasive surface. These cups and discs are mounted on mandrels (Fig. 4.6). For final polishing bristle brushes and rubber cups are used in conjunction with an abrasive paste; coarser abrasives such as pumice are used initially, followed by finer abrasives such as zirconium silicate, whiting or zinc oxide to produce the final

Fig. 4.6 Rotary instruments used in finishing and polishing.
From left: sandpaper disc and Moore's mandrel; cuttlefish disc and screw mandrel; finishing cup, incorporating abrasive, mounted on mandrel; bristle polishing brush and rubber polishing cup for use with abrasive and polishing pastes respectively.

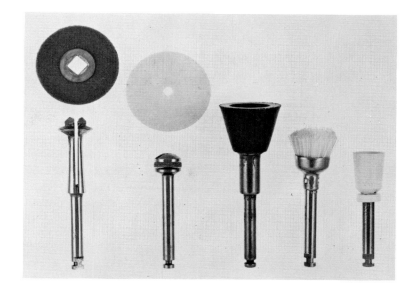

polish. Abrasive strips of varying grades are used to finish the approximal surfaces of restorations by hand.

EFFICIENT USE OF BURS

There are a number of simple guidelines which lead to the efficient use of rotary cutting and grinding tools, particularly burs.

● *Use as small a range of burs as possible* Where there are large numbers of burs from which to choose, time will be wasted finding a particular bur and removing it from the stand. On the other hand, with a small selection it is simple to find and remove the desired bur. Time-consuming bur changes will also be reduced if fewer burs are used for each operation.

● *Use each bur as few times as possible* Ideally, each bur should be introduced into the mouth a few times only during a cavity preparation and all work should be completed with it before changing to another bur. At first this may seem difficult but it will become simpler as the student's confidence and experience increase. It is inefficient to use a bur on a number of separate occasions when one planned use may be sufficient.

● *Use the most efficient shape of bur* If a rotating bur is held at a constant axis and moved around the walls of a cavity it will impose its shape on the cavity. In Fig. 4.7 a long pear tungsten carbide bur is being used to prepare an occlusal cavity for a plastic filling. If

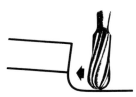

Fig. 4.7 Lateral cutting with a long pear bur produces a cavity with rounded internal angles and slightly undercut walls.

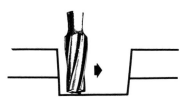

Fig. 4.8 Lateral cutting with a tapered fissure bur produces a cavity with square internal angles and slightly divergent walls.

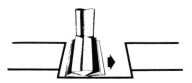

Fig. 4.9 Lateral cutting with an inverted cone bur produces a cavity with undercut walls.

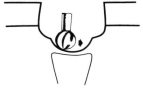

Fig. 4.10 A large round bur is more efficient and safer than a small one for excavating carious dentine. It cuts best when used with a lateral action. Note that the floor is not flattened otherwise the pulp may become involved.

held at a constant axis, this bur will produce sufficient undercut for axial retention and will give the rounded internal angles which are generally desirable in such a cavity. Similarly, in Fig. 4.8, a tapered fissure bur is being used to prepare a cavity suitable for an inlay. If held at a constant axis, this will produce walls having the required angle of divergence. In the same way an inverted cone bur can be used to produce undercuts with sharp internal angles (Fig. 4.9). In each of these cases the bur will produce the required shape as simply as possible. It is desirable to practise moving a stationary bur around a tooth until this can be done without any alteration in the axis of the bur, rather like moving a surveying rod around a study cast. Since caries tends to spread on a rounded front, it is most efficient to use a round bur to remove it (Fig. 4.10). The round bur is also less likely to expose a pulp horn, whereas the use of a fissure or inverted cone bur could bring the cavity dangerously near to the pulp. Some burs, such as the dome-ended fissure, perform a dual function; the tip is used for penetration and the side for lateral cutting.

● *Use the most efficient size of bur* If a large round bur is used to remove an extensive area of carious dentine (Fig. 4.10) it cuts rapidly and efficiently, yet the size of the bur prevents it from penetrating deeply at any one point. If a small round bur were to be used, the removal of caries would be slower and there would also be a greater possibility of penetrating too deeply. Modern teaching recommends that sound tooth substance should be preserved and cavities made as small as possible. Thus very fine fissure burs are used for extending occlusal fissures.

● *Use the bur with the most efficient surface* The most efficient cutting surface for a bur is that which produces rapid tooth removal and simultaneously gives a good finish to the walls and margins of the cavity. It is generally best to use plain-cut tungsten carbide burs run at high speed in cavity preparation as these produce a more precise shape, a smoother finish to the walls and less chipping of the margins than diamond or steel burs. Diamond burs are valuable for superficial cutting of enamel as in crown preparation and in the removal of amalgam fillings, but in cavity preparation they tend to give a rough surface finish to the walls with chipping of the cavity margins.

● *Use the most efficient speed range* For the initial entry into enamel and for the gross shaping of the cavity an air-turbine handpiece operating at speeds in excess of 300,000 r.p.m. should be used. For the removal of carious dentine a large round 'excavating' bur should be used at slow speeds of the order of 1500 r.p.m. A bur used for the precise finishing of internal surfaces and

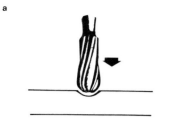

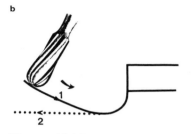

Fig. 4.11 (*a*) A long pear bur does not penetrate enamel efficiently when used with an end-cutting action. (*b*) It should be used with a lateral-cutting action, cutting obliquely to the required depth (1) and then horizontally (2).

margins of cavities should be used at 3000 r.p.m. At these lower speeds water cooling is not required.

● *Use the most efficient technique* A large round bur should be used with a sideways motion in the removal of carious dentine (Fig. 4.10). Examination of such a bur will reveal that the blades are deeply cut on the sides but shallow at the end of the bur. Further consideration will show that for a constant rotational speed, the blades on the sides have a greater linear speed than those at the end. Axial pressure on a bur may damage the bearings in the head of a handpiece and coolant spray may not reach the tooth. It follows that cutting with the side is more efficient than cutting with the end, so such a bur should be used with a sideways movement where possible. A long pear bur which is used to penetrate enamel should be used with a side-cutting action rather than an end-cutting action for the same reasons (Fig. 4.11). In order to prepare a cavity of even depth in relatively sound enamel and dentine, the bur is entered sideways into the surface of the tooth and gradually swung into an axial position as it penetrates to the correct depth. It should then be moved back across the cavity at the required depth so that with care it is possible to cut the general shape of a simple cavity with only two movements. Always try to establish the required depth as soon as possible and cut across at this level. This is more efficient than the gradual reduction of the tooth at a number of different levels and helps to keep the bur at the correct depth. The length of the cutting part of the bur can serve as a guide to the depth. If the cutting part is 4 mm long and a cavity depth of 2.5 mm is required, the bur should enter the tooth to about two-thirds of the length of its blades.

The same technique can be applied in the reduction of cusps. Cusps should not be reduced by gradually wearing the tooth down from the surface; instead it is better to enter the bur sideways into the surface to be cut until it reaches the correct depth. Several depth cuts may be made, using a bur of appropriate diameter, thus acting as a guide to the depth of the tooth substance removed.

If these seven rules are put into practice conscientiously they will eventually form an integral part of a sound operating technique. The inexperienced operator should realise that frequently he may not be able to see the part of the bur which is actually cutting. Instead he must form a mental picture of what is happening by observing the position and the angle at which the bur enters the cavity and the depth to which it has penetrated and by obtaining feedback through his sense of touch (kinaesthesis). When developed this sense will enable him to judge whether he is cutting sound enamel, sound dentine or carious dentine. It is simpler to make this judgement when using a hand instrument.

The operator should remember that burs are capable of damaging soft tissues and adjacent sound tooth surfaces. Adequate finger rests should be used with protection of the soft tissues by a tongue guard or mirror. Burs should be allowed to stop before removal from the mouth.

Hand instruments

Hand instruments may be manufactured from high-grade carbon steel or from stainless steel. Carbon steel is harder and can be sharpened to a better edge, but is subject to rusting and corrosion and so needs to be sharpened frequently. Stainless steel does not rust or corrode but produces a less satisfactory edge. The best, though initially the most expensive, cutting instrument is manufactured from stainless steel with a tungsten carbide insert to provide the cutting edge. These have a longer life than steel instruments and need sharpening much less frequently but, since tungsten carbide is brittle, they need to be handled with care to avoid fracturing the cutting edge.

DESIGN

Hand instruments are composed of three parts: the handle or shaft, the shank and the blade. Many hand instruments are double-ended giving either a right and a left form of the instrument or a large and a small form.

Handle   The handles of most instruments are octagonal and have serrations to prevent slipping. On one of the eight sides, serrations are absent and the number of the instrument, and in the case of cutting instruments the instrument formula, is inscribed. The instrument formula usually consists of three numbers; the first represents the width of the blade in tenths of a millimetre, the second the length of the blade in millimetres and the third the angle between the blade and the long axis of the handle in tetragrades (100 tetragrades = 360°). Occasionally a fourth number is given, indicating the reflex angle in tetragrades between the cutting edge and the axis of the handle; this is inserted between the first and second numbers in the instrument formula, thus the formula for one instrument is 20 95 9 12. Some instruments are supplied with larger light-alloy handles to improve the grasp and some of these have facets shaped to receive the fingers and thumb.

Table 4.1 Classification of hand cutting instruments (names from British Standard 2965 : 1958)

Name	Type of cutting edge	Angle of cutting edge to blade	Type of blade	Relation of cutting edge to angulation of shank (Fig. 4.14)	Angles in shank
Straight chisel	Single bevel straight	90°	Straight		None
Angle chisel	Single bevel straight	90°	Straight	East–west	1 (hoe) or 2 (contra-angle)
Hatchet	Single or bi-bevel, straight	90°	Straight	North–south	1, 2 or 3
Margin trimmer	Single bevel straight	60° and 120°	Curved	North–south	2
Excavator	Single bevel curved		Spoon, disc or pear		1, 2 or 3

Shank This connects the handle to the blade and is generally rounded in section, tapering to a narrower diameter where it joins the head. Sometimes the shank is straight, but more commonly it has one, two or sometimes three angles. Often two angles are used to set the blade at an angle to the handle and yet bring the working point into line with the axis of the handle, like the bur in a contra-angle handpiece, providing greater control and less tendency for the instrument to rotate in the operator's hand. On occasions, instruments with a single angle, although not so well balanced, are necessary to reach less accessible cavities.

Blade Hand cutting instruments may be divided into two groups, those with a straight cutting edge which are known as chisels and those with a rounded cutting edge which are known as excavators. Most chisels have straight, flat blades but in some cases, such as margin trimmers, the blade is curved and designed to be used with a lateral scraping motion. Double-ended cutting instruments have blades at each end, sharpened on opposite sides for use on opposing surfaces of a cavity.

TYPES OF INSTRUMENTS

Chisels Chisels are hand cutting instruments with a straight cutting edge. They may be divided into three groups (Table 4.1).

Fig. 4.12 Hand cutting instruments. *From left:* contra-angle chisel, hatchet chisel, two gingival margin trimmers and two spoon-shaped excavators.

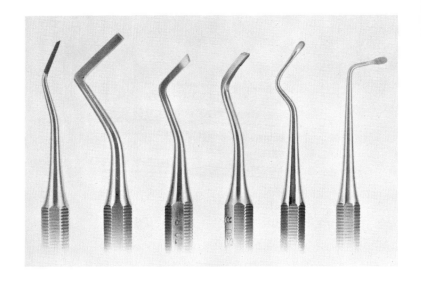

The straight chisel has the handle, shank and blade in a straight line. The angle chisel has one or two angles in its shank so this group may be divided into monangle chisels or hoes, and contra-angle chisels (Fig. 4.12). The angles do not lie in the same plane as the cutting edge but generally at right angles to it (Fig. 4.13, E–W). The hatchet is either mono-bevelled or bi-bevelled, has one or more angles in the shank of the instrument, the angles lying in the same plane as the cutting edge rather like the household implement of the same name (Fig. 4.13, N–S). The margin trimmer is similar to a mono-bevelled hatchet but has a curved blade, the convexity of which lies on the same side as the bevel of the cutting edge. It may be used to flatten the floors of approximal boxes, bevel gingival margins or prepare reverse bevels on gingival floors (Fig. 4.14).

Excavators These are hand instruments, usually double-ended, used for removing soft materials such as carious dentine from cavities and for trimming linings. The spoon-shaped excavator is the most commonly used design and has an oval-shaped blade with one concave and one convex surface meeting at a sharp cutting edge (Fig. 4.12). The disc-shaped excavator has one flat and one convex surface meeting at a sharp cutting edge. An excavator may be used with a forwards or sideways cutting motion and, because of its convex under-surface, the blade is prevented from penetrating too deeply. There is available a range of sizes of

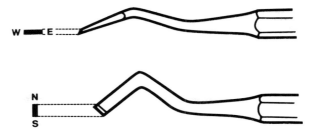

Fig. 4.13 Relationship of the cutting edge of a chisel to the plane of the angles of its shank.
(*Top*) a contra-angle chisel and (*bottom*) a hatchet chisel.

blade and of configurations of shank designed to reach different areas of the mouth.

Probes   These are single- or double-ended instruments which have a long, thin round-sectioned blade ending in a sharp point. They are available with a large variety of angles and curvatures (Fig. 3.1). The pocket-measuring probe is a specialised instrument graduated in divisions of two or three millimetres and having a blunt end; its function is to measure the depth of the gingival sulcus.

Condensers, plastic-filling instruments and carvers   Condensers are double-ended instruments for packing cement or amalgam into a cavity. The ends are at an angle to the handle. Some ends are cylindrical with a flat face (Fig. 4.15) while others are lozenge-shaped with a rounded or flat face. The flat face should be plain, not serrated, since serrations are difficult to keep clean. One end of the instrument is smaller than the other.

Plastic-filling instruments have flat elongated blades with rounded outlines (Fig. 4.15). They are usually double-ended, the plane of the blade at one end being in line with the handle (N–S) and at the other end at a right angle to the handle (E–W). They are used in the insertion, manipulation and shaping of plastic filling materials such as cements, aesthetic filling materials, amalgam and wax.

Carvers have flat blades with comparatively sharp edges and are used for carving amalgam or wax (Fig. 4.15).

Mouth mirror   This consists of a replaceable plane circular mirror attached to a shank and handle (Fig. 3.1). A disadvantage of the conventional type mirror is the possibility of a double image since the reflecting layer is on the back of the glass; this has led to the introduction of mirrors which reflect from their front surface only.

When working with the mirror, movements appear to be

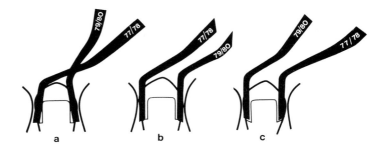

Fig. 4.14 Use of gingival margin trimmers (*a*) for flattening gingival floors and margins, (*b*) for bevelling gingival margins and (*c*) for placing reverse bevels. The instrument numbers are from the Ash catalogue; the instrument formula for 77/78 is 15 95 8 12 and for 79/80 is 15 80 8 12.

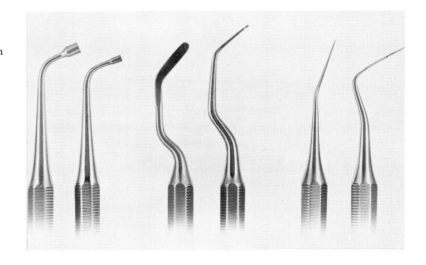

Fig. 4.15 Hand instruments for use with plastic materials.
From left: amalgam condenser (both ends), plastic-filling instrument (both ends) and Ward's No.1 carver (both ends).

reversed so that some practice is required to learn the technique of indirect working. Mirrors are also useful for retracting the cheeks or lips, in percussing teeth and in testing tooth mobility.

INSTRUMENT HOLDS

The student should learn to use the correct method of holding instruments from the beginning of his course. This is particularly important during preclinical work on the phantom head where it is possible to adopt methods which would be unsatisfactory in the mouth of a patient.

The method of holding a hand instrument or handpiece should give precise control and allow the required degree of power to be used with absolute safety. The operator must also receive as much feedback as possible during the use of the instrument; the patient

Fig. 4.16 Pen grasp used on upper left quadrant (*above*) and lower left quadrant (*below*). Note the finger rests on the teeth of the same arch.

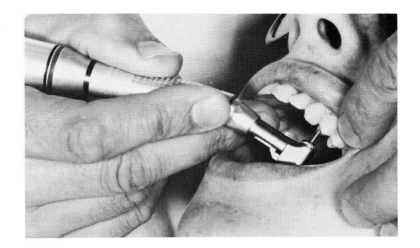

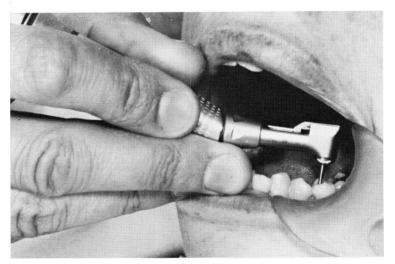

should feel complete confidence in the operator's ability to use the instrument safely and should not suffer discomfort.

One essential feature of good instrumentation is the use of a rest to steady the hand and provide a fulcrum for the movement of the instrument. Generally, the rest should be on a tooth, or several teeth, in the same arch since this provides a stable base. The rest teeth should be near to the tooth being operated upon particularly if some degree of force is being used. Sometimes a finger of the other hand may be used to provide secondary support. Occasionally it may be necessary to use the soft tissues as an auxiliary support but generally this is not desirable since they are unstable.

Fig. 4.17 Palm and thumb grasp used on upper right premolar (*above*) and upper right lateral incisor (*below*). Note the thumb rests.

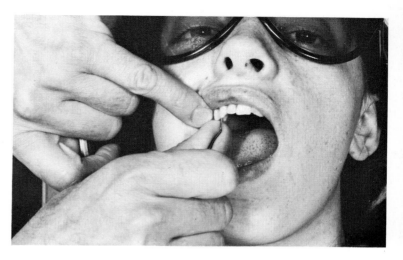

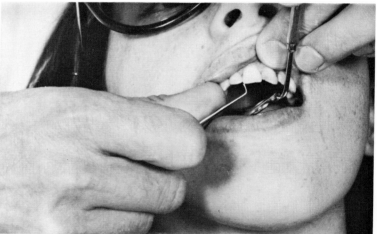

The rest may form a support for finger movements or, where more power is required, may form a fulcrum for arm and wrist movements. In the latter case the fingers are kept fixed, holding the instrument, and the whole hand is rotated about the fulcrum.

The most frequently used hold is the pen grasp (Fig. 4.16) which is very similar to the usual method of holding a pen. The second and, where there is space, the third and fourth fingers are used to provide a rest. The pen grasp can produce delicacy and precision of touch or a moderate degree of power. Sometimes a modified pen grasp is used where the second finger assists in holding the instrument and the third provides a rest. The pen grasp can be used with a movement away from the hand as with a chisel, towards the hand as with a scaler, or laterally as with an excavator or gingival margin trimmer.

The palm and thumb grasp (Fig. 4.17) is used occasionally on the upper teeth from the first molar forwards. The instrument is held between the palm of the hand and the fingers and is slid along the surface of the thumb which also acts as a rest. This grasp allows considerable power but provides less delicacy of control than the pen grasp. It is essential for the thumb to be positioned so as to resist the movement taking place without accidental slipping. When using a chisel, for example, on the occlusal surface of an upper tooth the thumb should rest mainly on this surface and not on the side of the tooth where it might slip. Force should never be used beyond the limits of safety and comfort; in fact since the introduction of high-speed rotary cutting, heavy force is rarely needed.

GUIDELINES FOR THE USE OF HAND CUTTING INSTRUMENTS

- Use only sharp instruments.
- Use the most suitable size of instrument.
- Use the instrument with the most suitable angle of shank and blade.
- Always keep the instrument under firm control so that there is no possibility of it slipping and causing injury to the soft tissues.
- Excavate deep caries away from the pulp. Excavation towards the pulp may lead to an unplanned exposure because of the transverse clefts which are present in carious dentine.

MAINTENANCE OF INSTRUMENTS

Modern handpieces are fine examples of precision micro-engineering. They are expensive and will repay careful maintenance with a longer working life. The manufacturers' instructions should be followed meticulously; generally they recommend the daily use of a cleaning and lubricating spray.

To be effective and safe, hand cutting instruments must be kept sharp. The sharpening process requires skill to maintain the designed bevel angle and to keep the cutting edge at the correct angle to the handle. Tungsten carbide tipped instruments are best returned to the manufacturer for sharpening. Steel chisels can be sharpened on a fine abrasive rotating wheel or reciprocating stone with guides for the different types of instruments. Care must be taken to remove only sufficient metal to produce a sharp edge, otherwise the life of the instrument will be shortened. Excavators

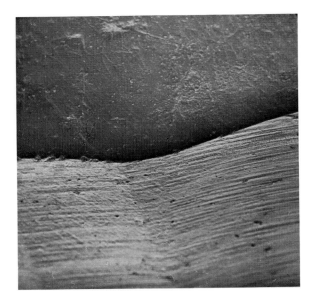

Fig. 4.18 Scanning electron micrograph of the occlusal margin of a cavity prepared with a plain-cut tungsten carbide fissure bur in an air turbine handpiece. The enamel surface is above and the cavity wall below. Note the fine grooves on the cavity wall and the slight chipping of the cavo-surface angle to the left.

must be moved in the correct path in contact with the revolving wheel to maintain their curved cutting edge. A flat Arkansas stone may also be used, but is slower and requires even more skill. Carbon steel instruments tend to corrode when wet-sterilised and require such frequent maintenance that they are less commonly used nowadays.

Surface finish produced by rotary and hand instruments

Research using the scanning electron microscope has provided much information about the surface finish produced by rotary cutting and grinding instruments and hand instruments during cavity preparation (Boyde & Knight 1970; Boyde *et al.* 1972). This information is important since it is generally believed that a cavity wall, and particularly a cavity margin, which is finished precisely to the shape demanded by the mechanical properties of the restorative material used, will produce the best marginal adaptation. In particular it is considered desirable to avoid cavity margins which are chipped, undermined or unintentionally bevelled.

When used in the turbine handpiece plain-cut tungsten carbide burs and Baker-Curson burs give the best finish (Fig. 4.18). In the approximal box of a cavity, where there is adequate access to approach the approximal surface with a fissure bur, one margin is known as the entry margin since the clockwise rotation means that

Fig. 4.19 Scanning electron micrograph of the occlusal margin of a cavity prepared with a diamond fissure bur in an air turbine handpiece. The scale is the same as Fig. 4.18. Note the deep grooving of the cavity wall and the gross chipping of the cavo-surface angle where enamel prisms have been fractured.

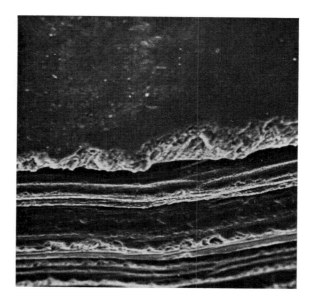

the blades are cutting into the tooth; the other is known as the exit margin since the blades cut out of the tooth. Entry margins can be given a nearly perfect finish but on the exit side burs with blades tend to fracture large chips of enamel out from the surface. Baker-Curson burs give a smooth finish to all margins.

Diamond burs used in the turbine handpiece produce deep horizontal grooving of cavity walls and floors with considerable chipping of the enamel at the margin of the cavity (Fig. 4.19). The degree of roughness of the finished surface depends on the size of the diamonds exposed on the surface of the instrument; large diamonds produce rapid cutting with a rough surface while fine diamonds produce a smoother surface with less rapid cutting. In approximal cavities, differences in finish exist between the entry and exit margins of the box. Entry margins tend to be neater while exit margins tend to show fracturing outwards of the surface enamel prisms. Diamond burs also cause some 'smearing' of the surface enamel.

Silicone carbide stones or finishing points used with water cooling produce a reasonably neat cavity margin. However, when they are run dry they tend to produce a 'welding' of tooth material, often at the enamel margins, resulting in an irregular finish. It seems likely that this is associated with heat production, but even when used with water spray some 'smearing' is produced.

Hand instruments tend to produce 'smearing' of the walls and margins. Even so, their use may be indicated where access for rotary instruments is restricted as in approximal boxes with limited extension.

Although most authorities teach that a well-finished cavity margin is desirable and that it might be expected that perfect margins would permit better adaptation of a plastic filling material with less micro-leakage, the limited evidence available indicates that this is not so. Menegale, Swartz & Phillips (1960) and Grieve (1971) found greater micro-leakage around restorations in cavities with smooth walls than in those with rough walls. Grieve, however, pointed out that greater marginal defects were visible in the latter case and considered that this was sufficient justification for producing a smooth marginal finish to cavities.

References

BRITISH STANDARD SPECIFICATION 2965 : 1958 for dental chisels, excavators, probes and scalers.
BOYDE A. & KNIGHT P.J. (1970) *Brit. dent. J.* **129,** 557–564.
BOYDE A., KNIGHT P.J. & JONES S.J. (1972) *Brit. dent. J.* **132,** 447–457.
GRIEVE A.R. (1971) *Brit. dent. J.* **130,** 239–242.
MENEGALE C., SWARTZ M.L. & PHILLIPS R.W. (1960) *J. dent. Res.* **39,** 825–835.
MORRANT G.A. & STEPHENS R.R. (1960) *Brit. dent. J.* **109,** 5–8, 42–46.

Chapter 5
Principles of cavity design and restoration

Good cavity design has been exemplified for many years by 'classical' cavities which proved to be satisfactory when teeth were in an ideal relationship to each other and when minimal amounts of caries were present. Memorising the shape of such cavities will not of itself produce a sound understanding of cavity design, particularly since many carious lesions do not fit within the 'classical' pattern. It is the comprehension and application of the principles embodied in these cavities which lead to the satisfactory preparation and restoration of teeth in the typical and the atypical situation alike. Each carious lesion should be viewed as posing an individual problem and the design of the cavity approached in a logical manner by:

● Defining the problem, that is, examining the tooth in detail and considering the possibility or desirability of restoring it.
● Establishing the methods by which the principles of cavity preparation can be applied to the treatment of the lesion.
● Arriving at a final design for the cavity.

Definition of the problem

The general nature of the restoration for a particular tooth will have been decided at the treatment planning stage and some information should have been collected regarding:

● Functional importance and occlusal relationships of the tooth.
● Aesthetic value of the tooth.
● Extent of the caries in the tooth from clinical and radiological evidence.
● Condition of the pulp.
● Effectiveness of the patient's oral hygiene.
● Health of the periodontal tissues.

These factors should be reconsidered in more detail before deciding on the type and extent of the restoration required.

Principles of cavity preparation

These can be summarised as:

- Provision of access.
- Removal of caries and tissue weakened by caries.
- Production of a biologically satisfactory shape.
- Production of a mechanically satisfactory shape.

It must be emphasised that these are underlying objectives and not necessarily stages to be carried out in a particular sequence.

PROVISION OF ACCESS

The establishment of access to allow removal of carious dentine by the cutting away of the overlying enamel must, in most cases, be the primary objective, but access must also be obtained for other reasons. It is needed for light and vision because, unless all points within a cavity can be examined visually, it is difficult to determine whether all caries has been removed and the correct shape produced. Access must be gained for all forms of instrumentation, and for coolants where high-speed cutting is indicated. Finally, access must allow lining and filling of the cavity. Early and rapid provision of adequate access is one of the most effective measures which can be taken to improve the quality and efficiency of cavity preparation, for inadequate access inevitably produces an inefficient operating technique and an unsatisfactory cavity.

REMOVAL OF CARIES AND TISSUE WEAKENED BY CARIES

Good cavity design must incorporate the removal of all, or virtually all, caries as this is usually the reason for preparing the cavity. It is the position and extent of the caries in the tooth which governs the basic form and approach to the cavity. The design must provide for the removal of all caries at the periphery of the tooth, particularly the enamel–dentine junction. The only residual caries which may be permitted is a very small amount immediately adjacent to the pulp in the technique known as indirect pulp capping (Chapter 12). The colour of the dentine, particularly in teeth which have been restored previously, is not an adequate single criterion by which to judge caries. The use of dyes to differentiate between tissue requiring removal and that which does not has been suggested (Fusayama 1980), but is not widely accepted. The most reliable clinical guide to the degree of demineralisation of the tissue is its hardness as tested by the feel of the dentine to pressure from a sharp probe or excavator. Once the caries has been removed the cavity must be inspected very carefully to ensure that the dentine barrier between the cavity and the pulp is still intact and that the pulp is not exposed.

Following this inspection any enamel or dentine not actually affected by caries but which can be seen to be too weak to form a useful part of the preparation should be removed. It is only when this has been completed that the operator will finally know the extent of the sound tooth substance available to support and retain the restoration.

PRODUCTION OF A BIOLOGICALLY SATISFACTORY SHAPE

This relates to those aspects of cavity preparation which contribute to the maintenance of the tooth in a healthy condition. The foremost of these is extension for prevention of recurrence of caries which was a tenet of good cavity design for many years. Equally important, but possibly less frequently considered, is the relationship of the cavity to the pulp chamber.

Extension for prevention

This means that the margins of a cavity should be extended into areas where caries is unlikely to occur. Cavity margins have been traditionally placed in areas which are readily cleansed by toothbrushing (Chapter 1), but this has tended to produce rather large cavities which may weaken the tooth. It is now believed that the patient's age, diet, oral hygiene and previous caries experience, that is their *caries preventive status*, should influence the degree of extension. This produces considerable variation in cavity outline and makes description of a typical cavity difficult. In general, the cavity designs described in this text relate to conventionally extended cavities with comment on how more minimal cavities may be produced when the patient's caries preventive status permits.

On the *occlusal surface* the cavity should include all the deeply cleft fissures of any fissure system which are thought likely to be affected by caries during the life of the restoration. The deeply cleft fissures are those which separate the major cusps, not the shallower grooves which occur within the cusps. Where a major anatomical feature, such as the oblique ridge of an upper molar, divides the fissure system into two distinct parts it may be wise to confine the cavity to one side of this. Where a patient has had a low incidence of caries for a number of years and the fissure systems of

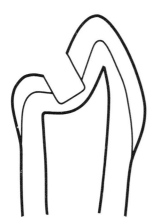

Fig. 5.1 Bucco-lingual section through a lower first premolar showing positioning of an occlusal cavity to avoid the buccal pulp horn in a young tooth.

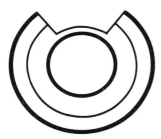

Fig. 5.2 Cross-section of a gingival cavity in a young premolar showing curvature of the floor to avoid the pulp.

the posterior teeth have remained mainly sound, full extension of the cavity is neither necessary nor desirable.

Where approximal surfaces are involved the gingival margin of the cavity need only be sufficiently clear of the contact area to ensure removal of caries and allow a matrix band to be placed. If interdental flossing is carried out effectively so that plaque never accumulates for more than 24 hours, all the margins can be similarly placed just clear of the contact area. Where accumulations of plaque persist, extension buccally and lingually into more readily cleansible areas is indicated. Whilst this part of the cavity is being prepared great care must be taken not to damage the surface of the adjacent tooth with hand or rotary instruments. Such damage produces a biologically undesirable situation for it both penetrates the surface layer of the enamel, which is more resistant to carious attack than the sub-surface enamel, and produces miniature stagnation areas in which plaque can form and grow undisturbed by oral hygiene measures.

On the *buccal and lingual surfaces* it is more difficult to apply the concept of extension for prevention. Few carious lesions develop in these surfaces occlusal to the line of maximum convexity, except for small isolated pit or fissure cavities. However, gingival to this line there are no areas in which the margins of cavities can be placed with complete confidence as plaque accumulates heavily in the whole of this area unless regularly removed. The precise shape of the cavity is dictated by the spread of the caries and by mechanical factors which will be discussed later. In these cavities it is better to replace the concept of extension for prevention with one of prevention by local preventive measures. Unlike the contact areas or the depths of the occlusal fissures these surfaces are readily accessible to improved oral hygiene procedures and the topical application of fluorides. It is measures of this nature that will ensure the longevity of gingival restorations rather than the precise outline of the cavity.

Relationship of the cavity to the pulp chamber

It may be necessary to modify the shape of a cavity to maintain an adequate thickness of dentine between it and the pulp chamber. An exaggerated bucco-lingual section through a lower first premolar (Fig. 5.1) illustrates the necessity for sloping the floor of a cavity in the occlusal surface of this tooth from the buccal to the lingual in order to avoid the large buccal pulp horn. Similarly, a transverse section through the cervical portion of a lower premolar in which a buccal cavity has been prepared (Fig. 5.2) shows that, if the cavity is to have adequate depth at the mesial and distal margins whilst not involving the pulp, the floor of the cavity must be curved in the same line as the outer surface of the tooth. Other examples of similar modifications are noted in the descriptions of specific cavities and restorations.

Sometimes two or more biological objectives conflict. Traditionally, it was considered desirable to place the gingival margin of a restoration below the margin of the free gingivae in the hope of protecting it from the recurrence of caries. More recently it has been shown that virtually all sub-gingival restorations encourage plaque retention and so irritate the gingivae, producing minor or even major periodontal problems. Such conflict is resolved where possible by compromise, in this case by placing the gingival margins of the cavities just clear of the contact area. These guidelines cannot, however, be applied where caries has progressed sub-gingivally.

PRODUCTION OF A MECHANICALLY SATISFACTORY SHAPE

This is concerned with preventing the displacement or fracture of the restoration. The effect of the cavity on the strength of the tooth must also be considered together with any additional concentrations of stress which may be produced by the restoration. This can be summarised as:

- Stability of the restoration

- Retention of the restoration $\left\{\begin{array}{l}\text{axial} \\ \text{lateral}\end{array}\right.$

- Strength of restoration $\left\{\begin{array}{l}\text{in bulk} \\ \text{at margins}\end{array}\right.$

- Strength of the tooth $\left\{\begin{array}{l}\text{in bulk} \\ \text{at margins}\end{array}\right.$

The terms stability and retention in relation to cavity design have specific meanings. All forces acting on a restoration can be resolved into components directed either towards the centre of the tooth or towards its periphery. The part of the cavity shape which resists displacement of the restoration by the components of force directed towards the centre provides *stability*, whilst that which resists displacement by the components directed towards the periphery provides *retention*.

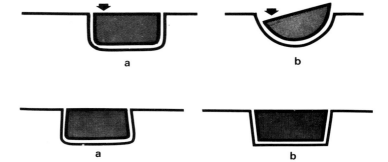

Fig. 5.3 (a) Definite walls and floors produce a stable restoration; (b) a saucerised cavity leads to an unstable restoration.

Fig. 5.4 (a) Filling in a cavity with internally diverging walls; (b) filling in a cavity with a slight taper.

STABILITY OF THE RESTORATION

If a cavity is to provide stability it must consist of clearly defined walls and floors at definite angles to one another (Fig. 5.3a). This does not mean that the actual line of junction between the walls and the floor must be a sharp angle; indeed in many cases it is better for the junction to be slightly rounded, but the cavity must not be a saucer-shaped depression. Fig. 5.3b illustrates how a force acting on one side of a restoration placed in such a saucerised cavity could rotate it out of the cavity. The shallower a cavity is in relation to its width the more clearly defined the walls and the floor have to be if instability is to be avoided.

RETENTION OF THE RESTORATION

If a restoration is to be satisfactorily retained within a cavity it must be able to resist displacement by forces which tend to pull it vertically out of the cavity (axial retention) and those which tend to force it out laterally (lateral retention).

Axial retention   If a parallel-sided piston fits closely the walls of a matching cylinder the force required to separate them would be very great. With restorations such perfect fit is not always achieved and it is wise, where possible, for a cavity to be made slightly narrower at its opening on the tooth surface than at its base (Fig. 5.4a). This is feasible when using materials which are inserted directly in a plastic state, such as amalgam, but where indirect restorations such as inlays or crowns are to be used this is impracticable. True parallelism would still give optimum retention, but it is usual for the preparations to be slightly tapered (Fig. 5.4b) to allow for operational variables.

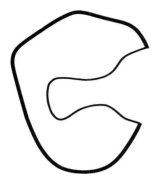

Fig. 5.5 An occlusal dovetail to provide lateral retention.

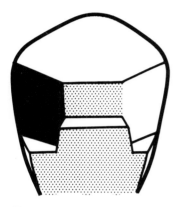

Fig. 5.6 Hemisected premolar tooth containing a mesio-occluso-distal cavity. The cavity is both narrower (bucco-lingually) and shallower in the centre than at either end.

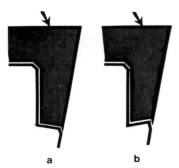

a   b

Fig. 5.7 (*a*) Unfavourably sloping; (*b*) favourably sloping gingival floors of inlay cavities.

Lateral retention In the single-surface cavity lateral forces are resisted by the walls of the cavity, but when one of these walls is missing, as in a mesio- or disto-occlusal cavity, some definite lateral retention must be provided. A common form of this is the dovetail (Fig. 5.5) where by using the occlusal fissure pattern of the tooth a positive mechanical lock is created which effectively prevents displacement of the restoration laterally in the direction of the missing wall. When both mesial and distal surfaces of the tooth are missing mesio-distal displacement of the restoration is prevented by the central portion of the cavity being narrower (bucco-lingually) and shallower than the approximal portions (Fig. 5.6).

The form of the gingival floor can also assist in providing lateral retention. If a force is directed from the occlusal surface on to a restoration with an unfavourably sloping floor (Fig. 5.7a) then the approximal section of the restoration tends to be displaced and stress produced at its junction with the occlusal section. A flat floor resists forces directed perpendicular to it, but not those directed towards the missing wall, whilst a favourably sloping floor (Fig. 5.7b) resists forces from both these directions. The favourable slope must be confined completely within the dentine as such a slope in the enamel would leave unsupported prisms at the cavity margins.

Pin retention When required pins may be placed in the dentine and a filling packed around them, or they may form an integral part of a cast restoration (Fig. 5.8). In the former case the pins may be angled in relation to each other to give greater axial retention. In the latter this is provided by the parallelism or near parallelism of the cast pins. In both cases the projection of the pins into the dentine and their association with the filling material provides additional lateral retention.

Extra-coronal retention The methods described so far for obtaining axial retention for cast restorations depend on the near-parallelism of internal cavity walls. However, axial retention can be similarly obtained between opposing external walls or between similarly opposing external and internal walls. A full crown, which covers the whole outer surface of the clinical crown of a tooth, obtains axial retention extra-coronally from the near-parallel opposing walls mesially and distally, and buccally and lingually.

Extra-coronal preparation can also aid lateral retention. For example, where there is an inadequate amount of tooth substance to prepare a dovetail for a disto-occlusal inlay, it may be possible to

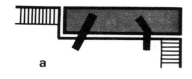

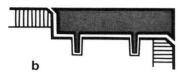

Fig. 5.8 (*a*) Pin retention for materials inserted in a plastic state; (*b*) pin retention for gold inlays. Compare the 90° angle at the margin of the cavity in (*a*) to the bevelled margin used with the cast restoration in (*b*).

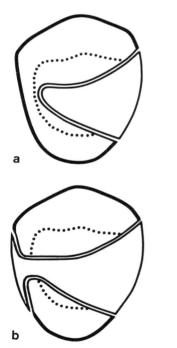

Fig. 5.9 Extra-coronal retention. (*a*) Restoration lacking lateral retention; (*b*) similar restoration with extra-coronal cast gold veneer providing lateral retention.

extend the casting in a thin layer or veneer to cover the mesial surface thus preventing distal displacement (Fig. 5.9). Extra-coronal retention cannot be used with plastic restorative materials, such as amalgam or composite, because of their inadequate physical properties.

Adhesion　At present there are no truly adhesive materials which can be used to restore posterior teeth in load-bearing situations. If, however, such a material is developed many of the techniques for providing mechanical retention in posterior teeth will become less important, as they have in anterior teeth with the advent of acid etch composites and glass ionomer cements.

STRENGTH OF THE RESTORATION

In bulk　A cavity must accommodate a bulk of restorative material sufficient to withstand any stresses likely to be imposed upon it. The design should also avoid the production of areas of stress concentration in the restoration. Photoelastic techniques of stress analysis have shown that the stresses created when a force is applied to a restoration are extremely complex (Graneth 1964a, b, c) but there appear to be two simple guidelines:

● In areas which are subject to stress a sufficient bulk of restorative material should be used provided that this is compatible with the biological and mechanical integrity of the tooth.
● Sharply projecting angles within the cavity should be avoided wherever possible.

At the margins　The margins of cavities are normally placed in enamel. This is a brittle structure and, unless firmly supported by dentine, will withstand little stress before cleaving along the line of the enamel prisms. These prisms lie at approximately 90° to the outer surface of the enamel and therefore the minimum permissible angle between the internal walls of the cavity and the external surface of the tooth is 90°. The high tensile and compressive strength of cast gold enables it to function satisfactorily in thin sections. The margins of a gold inlay cavity can, therefore, be modified to give a 135° bevel at the margin of the cavity; subsequently the marginal prisms will be overlaid with a thin layer of gold (Fig. 5.8b).

　　Amalgam and the aesthetic restorative materials are weak in thin sections and therefore the cavity must ideally be designed to produce a 90° angle at the margin (Fig. 5.8a). The resulting butt

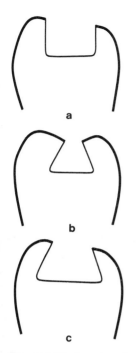

Fig. 5.10 Weakened tooth structure resulting from (*a*) excessive width of cavity, (*b*) excessive divergence of walls and (*c*) a combination of both.

joint is the most satisfactory compromise between the poor edge strength of these materials and the brittle nature of enamel.

STRENGTH OF THE TOOTH

In bulk   A natural concern for the strength and retention of the restoration can lead to the neglect of the physical properties of the remaining tooth substance. The necessity for avoiding unsupported enamel, that is enamel not supported by dentine, is well established, but it is frequently forgotten that reduction in width of a cusp will weaken it. The more load a cusp has to take the stronger it needs to be. It is only as strong as the thinnest section of tissue attaching it to the tooth, and tissue can be unnecessarily lost in two ways:

● By cutting away too much sound tooth tissue, as in the preparation of an excessively wide or deep occlusal cavity (Fig. 5.10a).

● By the use of too severe undercuts for the retention of the restoration (Fig. 5.10b).

These two may also occur at the same time and have an additive effect (Fig. 5.10c).

The width of the occlusal section of a cavity should normally not exceed one-quarter of the distance between the tips of the buccal and lingual cusps of the tooth. If it is essential for the cavity to be much wider than this then the cusps may need to be protected or modified. With a cast restoration it is possible to protect the cusps with gold and spread the occlusal stress evenly over the whole tooth. If only one of the cusps surrounding an amalgam cavity is unduly weak it may be possible to reduce the load it carries by grinding its surface, but where more than one cusp is involved a cusp-covered inlay is to be preferred.

Sharp angles within cavities should be avoided for, as well as their effect upon the restoration, they may act as areas of stress concentration within the tooth tissue and in many cavities they also project towards the pulp horns. Where practicable the angles between the walls and floors of cavities should be slightly rounded.

Localised areas of stress are also produced in tooth tissue by the provision of supplementary intra-coronal retention in the form of pins or screws (Courtade & Timmermans 1971). Such mechanical aids must be positioned with great care to ensure that they are placed firmly in dentine well away from both the enamel–dentine junction and the pulp.

At the margins   This has been discussed in relation to the marginal strength of the restorative materials.

75   *Principles of cavity design and restoration*

Terminology

At this point it is desirable to become conversant with certain basic terms which will simplify description and discussion of cavities. As in a room the surfaces within a cavity are known as *walls* and *floors*. It is necessary first to establish which surface in a particular cavity, is by convention, called the floor. The surfaces at right angles to this are known as walls. In a simple occlusal cavity the surface adjacent to the pulp is called the pulpal floor and the walls are named according to their position, that is, mesial, distal, buccal and lingual. In a cavity on the buccal surface of a tooth the surface adjacent to the pulp is known as the pulpal floor and the walls are then called mesial, distal, occlusal or incisal, and gingival. Compound cavities in posterior teeth which involve both the occlusal and approximal surfaces have at the base of their occlusal part a floor known as the pulpal floor and at the base of their approximal part a gingival floor; the wall connecting these two floors and adjacent to the pulp is known as the axial wall since it is parallel to the long axis of the tooth. The approximal part of such a cavity will also have a buccal and a lingual wall.

Where the outer surface of a tooth meets the prepared wall of a cavity a *cavo-surface angle* is formed. This is identified by using the name of the wall involved, for example, the mesial cavo-surface angle. The shape produced by the line of the cavo-surface angle on the external surface of the tooth is known as the *outline* of the cavity.

Where two surfaces meet within a cavity a *line-angle* is formed and this is identified by the names of the two surfaces involved, for example, the bucco-pulpal line angle. Where three surfaces meet within a cavity, as in the corner of a room, a *point-angle* is formed and is identified by the names of the surfaces involved. Finally, the term *axis* will be used to refer to a line at right angles to the floor or floors of the cavity.

The cavity classification originally devised by Dr. G.V. Black is still universally recognised and is based on the site of origin of the carious process.

Class I cavities are related to anatomical pits and fissures. They are most frequently found in the occlusal third of the crowns of molar and premolar teeth.

Class II cavities arise from the mesial and distal surfaces of molar and premolar teeth.

Class III cavities involve the mesial and distal surfaces of incisors and canines but do not involve the incisal edge.

Class IV cavities are similar to Class III but do involve the incisal edge.

Class V cavities commence in the cervical third of the buccal and lingual surfaces.

An alternative system of classification is the one which describes the surfaces of the teeth involved in the cavity, for example, mesial, distal, buccal, lingual and occlusal, or mesio-occlusal (MO), disto-occlusal (DO) and mesio-occluso-distal (MOD).

If these two systems are combined then more precise shorthand descriptions of cavities can be given, for example, Class III mesial, Class IV distal, Class V buccal, Class II DO and Class II MOD.

Selection of the restorative material

GENERAL FACTORS

General factors in the patient's background indicating or contra-indicating complex and expensive treatment have been discussed in Chapter 3, and these apply equally in the choice of restorative materials for individual cavities. If the oral hygiene is persistently poor or the prognosis of the tooth or the dentition is not good it is usually desirable to use simpler techniques and less expensive materials wherever possible. The choice of restorative material will usually be made at the treatment planning stage, but the local factors affecting the choice for the individual types of restoration can be better appreciated now that an understanding of some of the problems of cavity design has been acquired.

LOCAL FACTORS

Mechanical strength of the restorative material

An estimate must be made of the load which will be borne by the restoration. This will depend on the position of the restoration in a tooth, the relationship of the tooth to the adjacent and opposing teeth and additional factors such as the load of a denture rest or clasp on the restoration.

Mechanical strength of the tooth

Stresses similar to those applied to the restoration will be applied to the tooth. Gold may be chosen in preference to amalgam in order to cover and protect potentially weak areas of tooth tissue.

Appearance

If the restoration will be visible during normal functional movements of the mouth, the appearance of the restoration must be acceptable to the patient. If this choice conflicts with function, the problem must be carefully discussed and the possibilities of compromise explored, for example, in the choice of gold, porcelain or porcelain bonded to metal crowns.

Shape of the remaining sound tooth tissue

In some cases it may be clear that the use of a thin mesial veneer of gold to convert a DO into a MOD restoration would assist with a problem of retention. In others, the removal of undercuts to provide a satisfactory path of insertion for an inlay might require the removal of excessive amounts of sound tooth tissue and a filling material which could be inserted in a plastic state would then be indicated.

Special mechanical requirements

Cast gold restorations or porcelain bonded to metal crowns are indicated in situations where precision retainers for dentures are to be incorporated within a restoration or where it is desirable to alter the coronal contours of the tooth to receive a conventional denture clasp. They are also indicated where several restorations are to be joined together in the form of a splint or a bridge.

INDIVIDUAL RESTORATIONS

Class I

Amalgam is the most commonly used restorative material for Class I cavities. Cast gold is rarely used except perhaps where a number of more complex cast gold restorations are already required in one quadrant of the mouth and an additional occlusal inlay may conveniently be constructed at the same time. Currently, composite cements are regarded as unsuitable for the restoration of occlusal cavities, but where a small cavity exists in an otherwise sound occlusal surface it may be restored with an acid etch composite provided that the remaining fissures are sealed at the same time. As the physical properties of the composites improve they should be considered for use in larger cavities, but at present they have a particular use in the restoration of lingual access cavities in root-filled teeth.

Class II

Again, amalgam is the most frequently used material in this type of cavity. A cast gold inlay will, however, prove more durable, particularly for the larger restoration. In MOD cavities where there is moderate or extensive caries it may be advisable, particularly in premolars, to use a gold inlay with full or partial occlusal coverage to protect weakened cusps.

Class III

Composite cements are the materials of choice either as conventional filling materials or using an 'acid etch' technique. Glass ionomer cements have a limited use in areas where appearance is less critical. Cast gold inlays are occasionally used as a support for a bridge or a partial denture.

Class IV

An 'acid etch' composite restoration is now the most common solution. Where this is not practicable it is usual to proceed to a crown.

Class V

Amalgam is used for those restorations which are not normally visible. Composite cements are used where aesthetics are of primary importance and glass ionomer cements are particularly useful in the shallow irregular cavities left by toothbrush abrasion or root caries. Pin-retained gold inlays are sometimes used to receive gingivally approaching denture clasps.

Full veneer crowns

Where aesthetics are less important, i.e. molars and some premolars, gold is the material of choice as adequate strength can be provided with the minimum removal of tooth tissue. For anterior crowns aluminous porcelain provides optimum aesthetics, but requires more removal of tooth tissue. Porcelain bonded to metal is the technique of choice where good aesthetics are required but the incisor relationship, an unusual cervical contour or the inclusion of a rest seat preparation for partial denture dictates the use of metal in some part of the crown.

References

COURTADE G.L. & TIMMERMANS J.J. (1971) *Pins in Restorative Dentistry*, p. 10. C.V. Mosby Co., St. Louis.

FUSAYAMA I. (1980) *New Concepts in Operative Dentistry*, pp. 13–59. Quintessence.

GRANETH L-E. (1964a) *Odont. Revy.* **15,** 169–185.

GRANETH L-E. (1964b) *Odont. Revy.* **15,** 290–298.

GRANETH L-E. (1964c) *Odont. Revy.* **15,** 349–365.

Chapter 6
Linings, cements and dressings

Dentine physiology and sensitivity

There is strong evidence that the sensation of pain in dentine is associated with a movement of fluid in the dentinal tubules. Thus air-drying the surface of the dentine may result in an outward flow of fluid from the tubules as a result of capillary action (Brännström & Aström 1972). Cooling or heating the dentine surface or exposing it to reduced pressure or to chemicals which exert an osmotic effect also result in a flow of fluid with a sensation of pain. With a more severe stimulus there may be an associated aspiration of odontoblasts into the tubules and disorganisation of the odontoblast layer at the surface of the pulp. It is known that pain can be elicited by a cold stimulus before any change in temperature reaches the pulp; in other words, the surface of the dentine may react to the stimulus. Thermal stimuli, transmitted through filling materials of high thermal conductivity, such as metal, to the dentine surface, may result in pain and increased sensitivity to thermal changes. Matthews (1972) gives an excellent review of sensory mechanisms in dentine.

The combined effect of some materials and the bacteria present on the cavity floors can cause pulpal inflammation which may progress to pulpal necrosis. This topic will be dealt with at greater length in Chapter 12. Consequently, the dentist must be aware of the effects on the dentine and pulp of the materials used in conservative dentistry and he must take effective action to prevent damage to these tissues. The method most commonly used is to cover the dentine of the cavity floor, at least where pulpal irritation is deemed likely, with a material which does not irritate the pulp. Such a material is called a lining.

Linings

REQUIREMENTS OF A LINING MATERIAL

● It must be non-irritant to the pulp, unless the tooth is root filled or a non-irritant sub-lining has already been placed.

- It must have adequate strength.
- It must not react with the restorative material to be used.
- When set, it must be capable of being trimmed without crumbling or being dislodged.
- For use with metallic fillings, it should have a low thermal conductivity.

SELECTION OF A LINING MATERIAL

Linings can be divided into three categories: bases, liners and varnishes. Bases are materials used in relatively thick layers to replace lost dentine and to protect the pulp from chemical and physical irritants. Liners are aqueous or volatile organic suspensions of calcium hydroxide or zinc oxide which can be applied to a cavity surface in a relatively thin layer to protect the pulp from chemical stimuli. Varnishes are solutions of resins in an organic solvent and may contain small quantities of zinc oxide or calcium hydroxide. Low viscosity varnishes may be spread over the walls and floors of cavities to improve the marginal seal of restorations. Care is required in selecting the most appropriate material for use in a particular situation.

Bases

Modified zinc oxide–eugenol cements   These have been modified to produce a more rapid set and greater strength than is found in the simple zinc oxide and eugenol cement. They are harmless to the pulp and good thermal insulators; they handle easily and are moderately strong. They may be used in amalgam cavities, but not with acrylic resin or composite materials, as the eugenol acts as a plasticiser of the resins.

Ethoxybenzoic acid (EBA) cements   These are non-irritant to the pulp, are good thermal insulators, and are stronger than the modified zinc oxide–eugenol cements. When set they can be trimmed with rotary instruments without crumbling. They may be used in amalgam and inlay cavities and crown preparations. They should not be used with resin-based fillings as they contain essential oils which adversely affect these materials.

Polycarboxylate cements   These are slightly irritant to the pulp (Plant 1970). They are stronger than the EBA cements (Grieve 1969) and there is direct chemical adhesion to tooth substance, which is stronger to enamel than to dentine.

Zinc phosphate cements These are moderately irritant to the pulp and should not be used in deep cavities without a liner. They are good thermal insulators and have good handling properties. When set they are the strongest of these materials and can be trimmed with rotary instruments without crumbling. In general they have been superseded by the newer materials but where strength is required they may be used over a liner. They are also useful for the elimination of small areas of undercut in inlay cavities, provided that these are not near the pulp.

Liners

These materials are non-toxic to the pulp but are weak and relatively easily displaced. It has been suggested (Grajower *et al.* 1976) that some can inhibit the growth of micro-organisms present beneath restorations. They are the lining of choice for composite and glass ionomer cements and can be used beneath more toxic bases. With care they may also be used to protect the pulpal floors and axial walls of minimal depth amalgam cavities.

Varnishes

Some *in vitro* experiments have shown that the careful application of a varnish to the walls and floor of a cavity prior to placement of the restoration reduces marginal leakage and the formation of carious lesions on the internal walls of the cavities (Kidd 1976). Liners and varnishes also adhere more firmly to dentine than to composite filling materials, so that if the latter contract the dentine is still protected from bacteria and oral fluids which seep into the space (Grajower *et al.* 1976). More recent reports have drawn attention to the risks of increasing micro-leakage either due to the use of a varnish containing small quantities of CaOH and ZnO (Wilson & Smith 1978) or due to adverse interaction between varnishes and bases (Larsen *et al.* 1979; Yates *et al.* 1980). They may also pool and obliterate retention grooves (Wilson & Smith 1978) and clearly they must not be applied to enamel which it is subsequently intended to etch. At present varnishes cannot be unreservedly recommended for use in cavities. If they are to be used the agent of choice would be a simple low viscosity copal resin varnish, applied only to specific areas of the enamel and dentine, not to a base.

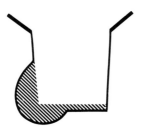

Fig 6.1 Cross-section of the occlusal section of an inlay cavity showing how lining material has been used to block out an undercut and also to line the floor.

Bases

The particular area of dentine that must be covered depends on the purpose for which it is being inserted. A base designed to prevent chemical irritation should cover the complete area of dentine from which tubules lead to the pulp. Where a base is designed to insulate against thermal change, it should cover those parts of the cavity where the thickness of the remaining dentine is considered inadequate to prevent the transmission of thermal changes to the pulp. Bases used to block out undercuts in inlay cavities should slightly over-fill all areas which are undercut in relation to the axis of withdrawal. The slight excess is trimmed back, after setting, to the required shape (Fig. 6.1).

Prior to mixing the material the cavity should be isolated and thoroughly dried; but it should not be dehydrated by the prolonged use of an air jet. The materials should be mixed according to the manufacturer's instructions and inserted without delay. The objective should be to place the cement only where it is required and in the correct thickness so that little or no trimming is needed. Although it has been traditional to complete the cavity preparation before placing the base this is not essential; it may be more efficient to place it as soon as all the caries has been removed. This will protect the pulp from additional trauma and any excess material can be removed during the final stages of cavity preparation.

Modified zinc oxide–eugenol and EBA cements For use in amalgam cavities these are mixed to a thick putty-like consistency. A small rounded mass of appropriate shape is positioned in the cavity with a probe and then moulded into shape using an amalgam condenser or plastic filling instrument which has been dipped lightly in cement powder to prevent sticking. Any gross excess is removed with an excavator, but should further adjustments be required they are best made with a bur after the cement has set.

Polycarboxylate cements This material, when used as a base, should be mixed to a thick putty-like consistency and applied as is described for modified zinc oxide–eugenol cements. Mixes which are too thick may give inadequate working time. Most operators use a separating medium such as alcohol to prevent it sticking to instruments (Friend 1969). Instruments should be cleaned immediately after use.

Zinc phosphate cement The powder is incorporated into the liquid in small quantities and the mix thoroughly spatulated between each increment to give a thick putty-like consistency. If the powder is added too quickly the material will tend to set rapidly on account of the exothermic reaction. It is handled in the same manner as an EBA cement.

Liners

These are applied with a special fine ball-ended applicator or the reverse surface of a small excavator. Just sufficient liner is collected on the head of the applicator, carried to the centre of the floor of the cavity and spread from this point without lifting the applicator from the floor. Further increments may be required but with practice it is simple to place these materials speedily and precisely.

Varnishes

A small piece of cotton wool held in a pair of tweezers is moistened with varnish which is then painted on to the surface of the cavity. The thin film of varnish is carefully dried with a gentle jet of air and the process repeated. Care must be taken to avoid any pooling of varnish within the cavity.

Cementing materials

Dental cements are used in the permanent placement of cast gold restorations. For this purpose they should have the following properties:

● They should be insoluble in oral fluids.
● They should adhere to dentine, enamel, porcelain and cast gold.
● They should be non-irritant to the dental pulp.

So far no cement completely fulfils either of the first two requirements. In the absence of true adhesion, retention is obtained by mechanical locking of the cement together with frictional retention.

The materials available are zinc phosphate, ethoxybenzoic acid and zinc polycarboxylate cements. These are essentially the same materials as those which are used in the lining of cavities, but they are mixed to a thinner consistency. There is also glass ionomer cement which is a modified version of the aesthetic restorative material.

Zinc phosphate cement   This has been in use for nearly a century and is the standard by which other cements are judged. It has no specific adhesion to the tooth or the restoration but forms a strong mechanical bond. When fully set it is almost insoluble in water, but is more soluble in dilute organic acids. It is irritant to the pulp and so a non-irritant base should be placed in deep cavities prior to the construction of an indirect restoration which is to be cemented with this material. This cement should be mixed carefully by the gradual addition of powder until a consistency is reached when a mass held up on a spatula will slowly slump off it.

Ethoxybenzoic acid cement   This causes little pulpal irritation and, when appropriately formulated, has a low solubility. It has no specific adhesion to the tooth or the restoration and forms a rather weaker mechanical bond than zinc phosphate. It can, however, be used to cement restorations on retentive preparations. Mixing of this cement requires care since, after an initial period of thickening, it becomes more fluid and further powder can be added until a consistency is reached similar to that recommended for zinc phosphate cement.

Zinc polycarboxylate cement   This adheres specifically to tooth substance but not to restorations unless the fitting surface of these has been plated with a base metal such as tin. Despite a low initial pH it does not cause serious pulpal irritation and its solubility is only slightly greater than that of zinc phosphate cement. With some brands the powder is mixed with one liquid for lining purposes and with another liquid when used as a cementing medium, so the correct liquid should be used. Surplus cement should be removed as soon as the initial set has taken place.

Glass ionomer cement   This also adheres specifically to teeth but not to conventional restorations. It does not cause serious pulpal irritation and should be mixed strictly according to the manufacturer's instructions. After placing the restoration, excess cement must be removed and varnish applied to the margin of the restoration to protect the cement.

Temporary restorations

Sometimes, for lack of sufficient time or from preference, a permanent restoration is not completed in a single visit. Construction of an indirect restoration, such as a crown or inlay, involves a period of time between the preparation and the insertion of the completed restoration. In these cases it is essential to insert a temporary restoration.

FUNCTION OF A TEMPORARY RESTORATION

- It should cover exposed dentine and prevent damage to the pulp and pain or discomfort to the patient. It follows that temporary cements should themselves be non-irritant.
- It should stay in position for as long as required but should be readily removable by the dentist.
- It should be well contoured and allow removal of plaque by the patient.
- It should prevent movement of the tooth or the adjacent teeth both laterally, by restoring the contact point, and occlusally, by restoring the centric stops. It should permit lateral and protrusive movements.
- It should restore a satisfactory level of appearance.
- It should permit continued function of the tooth.

SELECTION AND PLACEMENT

Intra-coronal preparations are usually filled with zinc oxide and eugenol cement. These make satisfactory restorations but may be tedious to remove. For inlay cavities the addition of cotton wool fibres into the mix can often allow it to be removed in a single piece, but this is not advisable with an amalgam cavity because of the undercuts. Where an amalgam cavity has been completed and temporarily restored, only the superficial part needs to be removed while the deeper part is retained as a base for the permanent restoration. If a temporary restoration is required to last some months the cavity may be filled with an EBA cement.

Extra-coronal preparations usually involve reduction of the occlusal surface, so there is a risk of the tooth moving occlusally between visits. This would spoil the completed restoration, and so it is necessary to plan a more careful temporary restoration of the occlusal surface. Stock temporary crowns, made from soft metal such as aluminium or silver-tin alloy, or from plastic such as polycarbonate, may be used, particularly for individual prep-

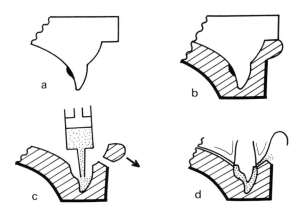

Fig. 6.2 Stages in construction of a temporary crown in the mouth. The explanation is given in the text.

arations. The crown form is selected with care and trimmed to fit along its gingival margin. This can be done with shears and trimmed with rotary abrasive instruments. The occlusion is similarly adjusted and the crown form cemented with a temporary cement. All surplus cement should be carefully removed.

Plastic crowns attached to thin wire posts are available for use with post crown preparations on anterior teeth. The length and angulation of the wire are adjusted to fit the prepared canal, the coronal section is trimmed and the crown cemented with temporary cement. A similar result can be achieved with a length of steel wire, hooked at one end. The wire may be stabilised in the root canal using soft wax and with the hook projecting from the canal but well clear of the opposing teeth. A hollow plastic crown form is then contoured, filled with auto-polymerising resin and seated in place over the wire. When the resin has set the crown, wire and wax are carefully removed and the margins and occlusion of the crown adjusted prior to cementing.

Where several crowns are being made at one time the use of individual crowns can be time consuming. It may be best to construct a matrix and use it to form the temporary crowns from quick-setting resin. The first stage is to replace any missing contour of the teeth to be restored, adding some additional contour in areas which are not in occlusion. This is done with wax on the cast (Fig. 6.2a). While the teeth are being prepared the cast is soaked in water and an impression taken of it in alginate material (Fig. 6.2b). After setting and removal, surplus alginate is trimmed away with a sharp knife. When the preparations are completed the impression is dried and a mix of resin, such as epimine resin, is injected into the area of the impression corresponding to the prepared teeth (Fig. 6.2c). The impression is seated in the mouth

(Fig. 6.2d) and after the resin has set it is removed. The surplus resin is trimmed away and the single block of temporary crowns placed with temporary cement. This technique has the disadvantage of not allowing interdental cleansing. Where there are several preparations not in alignment, the impression must be removed before the resin has completely set. After setting, the undercut areas within the crowns are trimmed back.

Temporary crowns can generally be removed by application of the edge of a strong instrument, using a fulcrum elsewhere in the same arch. Where temporary crowns appear to be very retentive at the fitting stage they should be eased to facilitate later removal.

References

Brännström M. & Aström A. (1972) *Int. dent. J.* **22**, 219–225.

Friend L.A. (1969) *Brit. dent. J.* **127**, 359–364.

Grajower R., Hirschfeld Z. & Zalkind M. (1976) *J. pros. Dent* **36**, 265–273.

Grieve A.R. (1969) *Brit. dent. J.* **127**, 405–410.

Kidd E.A.M. (1976) *J. Dent.* **4**, 199–206.

Larsen G.H., Moyer G.N., McCoy R.B. & Pelleu E.B. (1979) *Oper Dent.* **4**, 51–55.

Matthews B. (1972) *Proc. Roy. Soc. Med.* **65**, 493–495.

Plant C.G. (1970) *Brit. dent. J.* **129**, 424–426.

Wilson N.H.F. & Smith G.A. (1978) *Brit. dent. J.* **145**, 331–334.

Yates J.L., Murray G.A. & Hembree J.H. (1980) *Oper. Dent.* **5**, 43–46.

Chapter 7
Amalgam restorations

Dental amalgam was first introduced in 1826 as 'silver paste'. The early amalgam fillings were made of filings from silver coins mixed with mercury, but they were unpredictable materials and during part of the nineteenth century their use was declared by the American Society of Dental Surgeons to be malpractice. Later the physical properties of amalgam were investigated by Thomas Fletcher and John and Charles Tomes in England and by G.V. Black in the USA. The latter produced a silver-tin alloy which, when mixed with mercury, provided the first satisfactory plastic filling (Lufkin 1948). There has been a continuous improvement in the properties of amalgam alloys culminating in the development of the high copper alloys which do not contain the weak gamma 2 phase. These materials are stronger than and corrode less than their precursors. Dental amalgam as prepared for insertion in the cavity consists essentially of particles of alloy intimately mixed with sufficient mercury to provide a workable plastic material which begins to set after a few minutes. The plastic mass is packed into a suitably shaped cavity. It is pressed or vibrated so as to remove any excess mercury and bring the filling material into close apposition with the sides of the cavity.

Principles of cavity design for amalgam restorations

Two features in the physical characteristics of amalgam affect the design of cavities for use with this material:

● Amalgam is a material which when initially mixed is plastic and which subsequently sets hard, so that it can be placed into cavities whose shape provides positive mechanical retention.
● Amalgam has relatively low tensile strength and cannot be used in thin sections either within the main part of the restoration or at the margins.

The detailed application of the principles of cavity design will be related to the individual cavity preparations.

Fig. 7.1 Stages in the preparation of a Class I cavity.

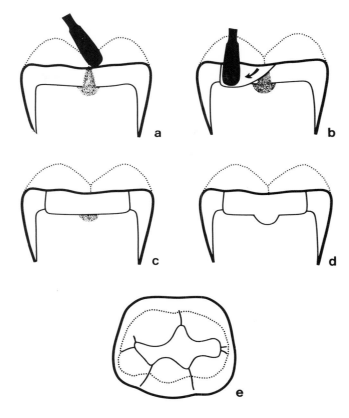

CLASS I

Access

Direct access is gained to the occlusal fissure system of a molar or premolar tooth using a long pear tungsten carbide bur in the high-speed handpiece. This bur has a round tip and a shape which will tend to produce the appropriate divergence of the walls towards the floor of the cavity. The tip of the bur is held immediately above the point of easiest entry to the occlusal surface, such as a point where obvious carious destruction has taken place or where there is some pre-existing restoration. The bur is held at 45° to the long axis of the tooth (Fig. 7.1) which enables the initial entry to be made with the side of the bur, as this cuts most efficiently. As cutting commences, the handpiece is rotated so that the bur comes to lie parallel to the long axis of the tooth. At this stage, the tip of the bur should have penetrated the enamel and be cutting just within the dentine. The deepest point

91 *Amalgam restorations*

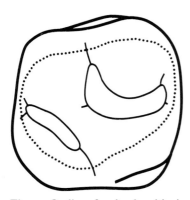

Fig. 7.2 Outline of occlusal cavities in an upper molar leaving the oblique ride intact.

of this cavity will be approximately 2.5 mm deep. Keeping the bur in the axis of the cavity it is traversed along the fissure system so as to produce a flat-floored groove from just within the mesial to just within the distal marginal ridge, care being taken not to undermine either of these ridges. This groove is then widened bucco-lingually until there is adequate access for removal of caries and the insertion of the restoration. Where there is minimal fissure caries this should not exceed one-quarter of the intercuspal distance. Any deep fissures running towards the buccal or the lingual margins of the tooth are included in a similar manner and the outline of the cavity is gently rounded.

When the patient has a good caries preventive status the outline of the cavity may be confined to those fissures showing evidence of caries. Where a major anatomical feature such as the oblique ridge of an upper molar or the transverse ridge of a lower first premolar divides the fissure system into two discrete parts, the cavity may be confined to one side of the ridge only (Fig. 7.2). If, however, caries has encroached upon the dentine supporting such a ridge the cavities should be joined.

Removal of caries

Where only a moderate amount of caries is present it will be found that the cutting of this basic outline removes it. If caries is observed under the cusps it is necessary to extend the margins of the cavity further up these cusps until adequate access to all caries can be obtained. Once the basic outline of the cavity is established any remaining caries is removed either with excavators or with a large round bur rotating at a slow speed. All caries is removed from the periphery of the cavity with particular attention being paid to the enamel–dentine junction. Dentine which feels soft to a sharp excavator is removed from the floor of the cavity unless pulpal exposure is likely in which case indirect pulp capping (Chapter 12) may be considered.

Biological and mechanical form

In a simple cavity this is usually produced whilst providing access and removing caries. The margins of the cavity will have been extended to include the parts of the fissures which are most difficult to cleanse with a toothbrush and deep fissures will have been removed.

The cavity has a generally flat floor to provide stability, and slightly undercut walls to provide retention, whilst the line angles

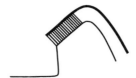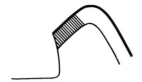

Fig. 7.3 Occlusal cavo-surface angle: (*left*) incorrect, (*right*) correct.

between the floor and the walls are slightly rounded. Where caries has extended more than 1 or 2 mm into the dentine no attempt should be made to flatten the floors of deeper cavities, as this would be likely to result in pulpal damage or exposure (Fig. 7.1).

All weakened or unsupported enamel prisms should be removed from the margins of the cavity. A good finish to the margin is produced by a plain-cut tungsten carbide or Baker-Curson bur rotating at high speed. Ideally, a 90° cavo-surface angle should be produced but, in view of the angulation of the cusps, it is frequently found that a rather more obtuse cavo-surface angle results and angles of up to 110° are considered acceptable (Fig. 7.3).

Summary

The essential features of a fully extended Class I amalgam cavity can be listed as:

● The cavity includes all deep fissures.
● The margin of the cavity is placed approximately one-quarter or less of the way from the base of the fissures to the tip of the cusps, unless otherwise dictated by the spread of caries.
● There is an internal divergence of the walls of the cavity, particularly on the buccal and lingual sides, so that the cavity is wider at the pulpal floor than where it meets the surface of the tooth.
● Care is taken not to undermine the mesial and distal ridges.
● The floor of the cavity is situated entirely within the dentine. The cavity will therefore be at least 2.5 mm deep.
● The line angles between the walls and the floor are slightly rounded.
● The floor is essentially flat, but where caries extends more than 1–2 mm into the dentine, no attempt is made to flatten the floor by deepening the whole cavity; once caries is removed, sound dentine should not be disturbed.

93   *Amalgam restorations*

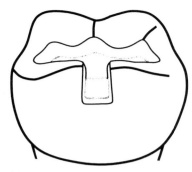

Fig. 7.4 Class I cavity with buccal extension.

CLASS I WITH EXTENSIONS

In molars, some fissures extend on to the buccal and lingual surfaces of the teeth. Where these fissures are carious it is necessary to make a small extension from the occlusal restoration through on to the buccal or lingual surface of the tooth (Fig. 7.4). This is carried out by taking a long pear bur along the fissure from within outwards. The depth of this extension should be that of a minimal occlusal cavity. In some cases this provides satisfactory extension, but frequently the fissure extends farther gingivally, so a small step is made from the occlusal floor into the extension. It is incorrect to attempt to cut out the whole of the occlusal floor at this increased depth as this will lead to unnecessary destruction of sound dentine. The width of any extension should be sufficient to accommodate the smallest available amalgam condenser.

CLASS II

Access

These cavities present a rather different problem to those of a simple occlusal cavity as in the majority of cases it will not be possible to have direct access to the carious surface. Access must be provided through some other surface of the tooth which may or may not be carious. The usual approach to approximal caries is through the occlusal surface of the tooth.

Biological form

The occlusal part of the cavity is extended in essentially the same manner as a Class I cavity. On the approximal surface of the tooth the gingival margin is positioned sufficiently clear of the contact area to ensure the removal of caries and to allow a matrix to be placed. The buccal and lingual margins may be similarly situated in patients with a good caries preventive status, but if this is poor these margins must be extended on to areas where they can be seen and cleaned by the action of a toothbrush. The cavity is not usually an even depth throughout but is designed with a step in the floor to minimise tissue destruction and avoid the pulp chamber.

Mechanical form

These cavities present problems because they are no longer simple and four-sided, the whole of one wall being missing.

Axial retention for the restoration is provided by the internally

Fig. 7.5 Correct buccal extension of the approximal box of a Class II restoration for a patient with a poor caries preventive status.

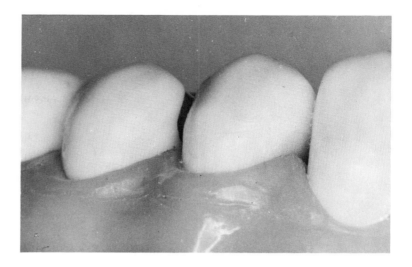

diverging form of the buccal and lingual walls of the occlusal section of the cavity and the divergence towards the gingival margin of the buccal and lingual walls of the approximal box.

Lateral retention Bucco-lingual displacement of the restoration is prevented by the buccal and lingual walls of the cavity. Mesio-distal displacement is prevented by a dovetail in the occlusal section of the cavity and possibly by the use of a favourably sloping gingival floor in the approximal box as discussed in Chapter 5.

A rounded pulpo-axial line angle increases the bulk of amalgam present at the junction of the occlusal and the approximal sections of the cavity, and reduces the undesirable concentrations of stress which occur at sharp line angles.

Marginal strength of both enamel and amalgam at the buccal and lingual borders of the approximal box is assured by careful shaping and positioning of these walls. Thin, weak sections of amalgam are produced if these walls are flared out and weak enamel margins can be produced by the removal of excessive amounts of buccal and lingual dentine. The correct form provides a 90° butt joint with adequate strength for both enamel and amalgam (Fig. 7.6). The greater the bucco-lingual width of the approximal box the more difficult it is to provide a strong margin for both enamel and amalgam simultaneously. Hence the emphasis on producing the minimum bucco-lingual extension compatible with the patient's caries preventive status. The development of modern designs for Class II cavities is well discussed by Rodda (1972).

95 *Amalgam restorations*

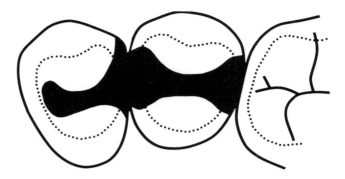

Fig. 7.6 Cavo-surface angles on the buccal and lingual aspects of approximal boxes: (*left to right*) greater than 90° with weak amalgam edges, less than 90° with weak enamel margins, correct 90° butt joint with conventional extension.

Preparation

Access to the occlusal section of a mesio-occlusal or a disto-occlusal cavity is gained in exactly the same way as for a Class I restoration, and the outline of the occlusal section is essentially similar. Where the approximal box is to be prepared the bur is taken farther approximately so that it cuts into and weakens the marginal ridge. The long pear bur is then positioned just within the weakened marginal ridge and a vertical slot is cut to the intended level of the gingival floor (Fig. 7.7d). In cutting the slot the bur is not only moved directly buccally and lingually but the handpiece is angled slightly so as to ensure that the gingival portion is slightly wider bucco-lingually than the occlusal. The remaining approximal enamel is broken down with a chisel (Fig 7.7e).

The preparation of the approximal box in this manner minimises the risk of damage to the adjacent tooth from the use of burs and ensures a minimal bucco-lingual extension. Where caries is more extensive, it is impossible to maintain an intact layer of enamel whilst preparing the approximal box and the inexperienced operator would be well advised to place a metal strip around the adjacent tooth to assist in protecting it from the bur. It is instructive to examine the marks on this strip when cavity preparation has been completed. In those cases where the spread of caries necessitates a wider box, the buccal and lingual margins may be prepared with a plain-cut tungsten carbide bur rather than a chisel. If adjacent approximal surfaces are carious, it is usually more efficient to prepare the cavities simultaneously.

Removal of much caries normally takes place during the basic cavity preparation but once the essential form of the cavity has been established any remaining caries is removed using large round burs and excavators.

Trimming of the enamel margins in the occlusal section is best

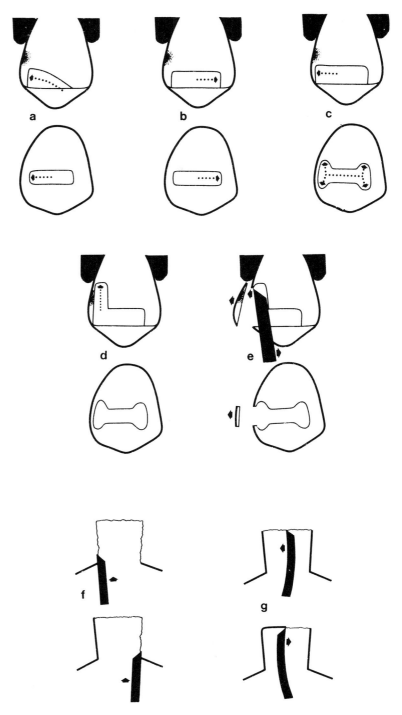

Fig. 7.7 Stages in the preparation of a Class II cavity. Details of the stages of preparation are given in the text.

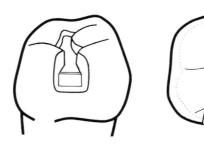

Fig. 7.8 Minimal Class II cavity in a molar.

carried out with a cylindrical Baker-Curson bur, but the margins of a minimal approximal box are better trimmed with hand instruments. The buccal and lingual margins are trimmed by planing with a hatchet or a contra-angle chisel (Fig 7.7f) whilst the gingival margin requires the use of a margin trimmer (Fig 7.7g). The latter is positioned with its cutting edge at right angles to the tooth surface and is then drawn along the margin removing any weak enamel.

A final finish can be imparted to the gingival margin with the flat end of a Baker-Curson bur. In larger cavities a similar bur may also be used to finish the buccal and lingual margins, but care must be taken to maintain a 90° cavo-surface angle and not to develop a small bevel.

The preparation of an MOD cavity is fundamentally similar to that of an MO or DO cavity except than an approximal box is placed at either end of the occlusal section of the cavity. The same basic biological and mechanical concepts apply except that lateral retention in a mesio-distal direction is provided by the vertical walls in each approximal box instead of by the occlusal dovetail. Buccal and lingual extensions may be required for Class II as for Class I cavities.

Summary

The essential features of a fully extended Class II cavity preparation can be described as:

● The occlusal section of the cavity is similar to a Class I cavity with a minimum depth of approximately 2.5 mm.
● The approximal box is normally in the form of a step down to the mesial or distal side of the pulp chamber.
● The buccal and lingual margins of the approximal box are placed so that they are just accessible to the cleansing action of a tooth brush.
● The gingival margin of the approximal box is placed so that

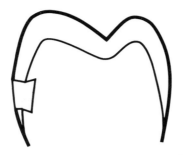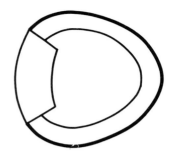

Fig. 7.9 Class V cavity in a premolar. (*Left*) Longitudinal section showing occlusal and gingival retention grooves; (*right*) cross-section showing curved floor and absence of mesial and distal undercuts.

there is a sufficient space between it and the surface of the adjacent tooth to place a matrix band.

● Axial retention is provided by making the buccal and lingual walls of the occlusal and approximal parts of the cavity diverge as they approach the floors.

● Lateral retention is provided by the occlusal dovetail (MO or DO), or the vertical walls (MOD).

● The axio-pulpal line angle is rounded.

● Space for adequate bulk of amalgam is provided.

The essential features of a minimal extension cavity are the same except that the extension of the cavity is limited to that which is necessary to remove caries and produce a satisfactory mechanical form.

CLASS V

Access

This is in most cases direct and easy through the partially demineralised tissue of the carious lesion.

Biological form

This is primarily concerned with maintaining the integrity of the pulp. A transverse section through the cervical portion of a lower premolar, in which a Class V cavity has been prepared (Fig. 7.9), demonstrates that if there is to be an adequate depth at the margins without involving the pulp, the floor of the cavity must be curved in the same line as the outer surface of the tooth.

In the gingival third of the tooth where these cavities occur there is no area in which plaque does not accumulate, if not regularly removed. Equally, all of this area is readily cleansable if reasonable tooth brushing habits are developed and so the precise size and shape of the cavity is dictated by the spread of caries and by mechanical factors.

Mechanical form

This is essentially that of a simple four-sided cavity but with the added complication of being curved around the tooth. This curvature is more marked in premolars and lower incisors than in molars and upper incisors. In the former group, the major problem is to provide retention without undermining the enamel margins. It is impossible to place undercuts mesially and distally, at least not without very considerable weakening of these walls (Fig. 7.9). There is less tendency for this to occur occlusally and gingivally so this is where the undercuts are placed. In molars and upper incisors the buccal surface is much flatter and, unless the cavity extends almost on to an approximal surface, undercut can be placed on all sides.

The smaller the outline of these cavities the easier it is to provide satisfactory retention and stability but, in view of their shallow form, sharp line angles are desirable to provide maximum retention and stability for the restoration. In this situation such line angles do not project towards the pulp and the stresses acting upon the surface are minimal, so sharp line angles may be employed without risk to the pulp or the fear that stresses within the tooth will weaken it under load. The enamel margin is finished to an angle of 90°.

Preparation

This consists essentially of the removal of caries and any remaining weak tooth tissue, together with the provision of retention. In these cavities the amount of tissue to be removed is small, precise working is required and virtually all the tissue to be removed has been to some extent softened and demineralised by the carious process. Conventional speed instruments are therefore more suitable than the air turbine. Entry is made into the tooth and caries removed with a moderate sized round bur. Using a plain-cut fissure bur held at 90° to the surface of the tooth, the walls of the cavity are squared up to produce a cavo-surface angle of 90° and a minimum depth of 1.5 mm is established. An inverted cone bur is used to produce small undercuts in the occlusal and gingival walls of the cavity. In molars or other teeth where the cavity is being prepared in a relatively flat surface the same bur may be used to introduce similar small undercuts in the mesial and distal walls. The enamel margins are gently trimmed with a cylindrical Baker-Curson bur.

Summary

These cavities appear simple to prepare but certain salient features must not be forgotten:

● If adequate mesial and distal depth is to be provided without involvement of the pulp, the floor of the cavity must be equidistant from the original surface of the tooth except where the extent of caries necessitates deepening a particular area.
● Owing to the shallow form of the cavity sharp line angles are indicated to avoid a saucerised cavity with poor retention and stability.
● Undercuts for retention must not be provided mesially and distally unless the tooth surface is relatively flat.
● Occlusal and gingival undercuts must be provided with caution as unsupported enamel is produced if extensive undercuts are created.
● The gingival margin of the cavity should be carried below the margin of the free gingivae only if this is necessitated by the spread of caries.
● The necessity for good oral hygiene in this area must be stressed to the patient as this is the most effective preventive measure in this region.

Final assessment

When cavity preparation is complete a thorough debridement is carried out. Any large particles of debris are removed with an excavator and the cavity is thoroughly cleansed with an air and water spray, dried gently with a jet of warm air and carefully inspected for faults. This inspection will occupy only a few seconds of an experienced operator's time but the student should carefully examine every aspect of the cavity in detail and assure himself that each objective of cavity preparation has been successfully carried out and that the cavity is as functional as possible.

Linings

The different types of cavity lining materials available have been discussed in Chapter 6. The primary function of a lining in an amalgam cavity is to prevent the transmission of thermal stimuli from the metallic filling to the sensitive dentine. In addition to having a low thermal conductivity a lining material for use with amalgam must have sufficient compressive strength to withstand

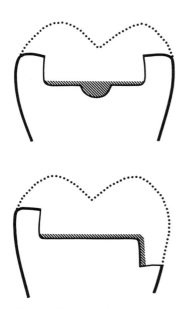

Fig. 7.10 Cross-sections of molar teeth showing the lining of (*a*) a Class I cavity with an irregular floor and (*b*) a Class II cavity.

the stress of amalgam condensation if it is not to be displaced when amalgam is packed into the cavity.

A layer of a base will normally be placed on the axial walls and the pulpal floors (Fig. 7.10). This layer need only be 0.5 mm thick to insulate the dentine and it should not be thicker than this in shallow cavities or it will significantly reduce the strength of the restorations. Indeed, in minimal depth cavities the base may be omitted and a thin layer of liner placed adjacent to the pulp. Care must be taken to ensure that the lining material does not obliterate any positive retention within the cavity. Liners and bases must never approach the cavity margins as all of these are more soluble in the oral fluids than amalgam.

There is no justification in amalgam cavities for attempting to restore a more ideal internal form to the cavity by inserting large amounts of base. Nevertheless, minor irregularities in the floor of the cavity may with advantage be obliterated whilst placing an adequate base (Fig. 7.10). All the bases currently available are weaker than amalgam and most of them do not bond reliably to dentine under routine clinical conditions. It is therefore unreasonable to expect that the replacement of lost tooth tissue with a base will improve the mechanical characteristics of the cavity. The necessary thickness of lining to insulate the pulp should be placed over the dentine and the remainder of the cavity filled with amalgam. Where cavities are very deep it may be expedient to use a somewhat thicker base, if this can be done without weakening the finished restoration, in order to reduce the time taken in condensing a very large quantity of amalgam and the cost of this material.

Amalgam technique

PROPORTIONING AND TRITURATION

In view of the hazards of handling mercury (Chapter 13) the traditional means of proportioning and triturating amalgam are no longer used; only sealed systems are now acceptable. The ideal method is to use commercially sealed pre-dispensed capsules containing the correct proportions of alloy and mercury in separate compartments within the capsule. When amalgam is required the capsule is momentarily compressed so that the mercury and alloy inside can mingle. The capsule is then placed in a mechanical vibrator for a precise time. This shakes the capsule violently so that the alloy and mercury are intimately mixed. The capsule is opened and the amalgam is ready for use. A less acceptable technique is to use a machine which contains separate refillable reservoirs for alloy and mercury. Movement of a handle dispenses volumetrically measured proportions of mercury and alloy into a trituration capsule which is firmly attached to the machine. Activation of a timing device ensures that this capsule and its contents are shaken violently for the required time. The capsule can then be detached and the amalgam used.

CONDENSATION

The objectives of condensing amalgam into the cavity are:

● To bring about the close approximation of the particles of material in the filling, removing any air spaces from the completed restoration.
● To bring the filling material into close contact with the walls of the cavity.
● To express any excess mercury from the mix.

Amalgam must always be condensed into a clean dry isolated cavity as moisture contamination of the material leads to a more friable porous restoration. Moisture contamination of dental amalgam produced with zinc-containing alloys leads to an excessive expansion of the material. This may result either in pain or in the restoration increasing in dimension so as to produce unsupported amalgam at the margins of the filling.

Small increments of amalgam are placed into the cavity and thoroughly condensed using either hand or mechanical condensers. The choice of technique will depend on the size and situation of the restoration as well as the type of alloy used. In general, the larger the restoration the greater the advantage in mechanical condensation. However, as alloys containing quantities of spherical particles tend to produce a very soft plastic mass when vibrated, hand condensation is indicated with such materials.

Hand condensation

This consists of alternately placing small quantities of amalgam in the cavity from an amalgam carrier (Fig. 7.11) and then thoroughly condensing. Each increment of amalgam is thoroughly condensed by heavy pressure from a suitably shaped condensing instrument. Each area pressed is overlapped by the next until the amalgam placed in the cavity is firmly condensed axially against the floor and laterally against the walls. Further increments of amalgam are then added and the stepping procedure is repeated

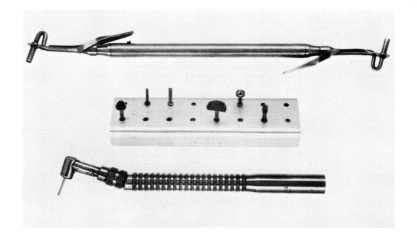

Fig. 7.11 (*Upper*) double ended amalgam carrier; (*centre*) selection of vibrator points in rack; (*lower*) Bergendal vibrator with small cylindrical point in position.

across the surface. When noticeable amounts of soft mercury-rich amalgam are brought to the surface this is removed and the cavity is incrementally filled until an excess of amalgam is present. During this condensation excess should be shaped to the general contours of the tooth (Fig. 7.12) which will improve the condensing of the margins and simplify the subsequent carving. It is essential in hand condensation to apply heavy pressure to the material and to apply this pressure repeatedly.

Where large cavities are being filled it is necessary to use several small mixes of amalgam to complete the filling. If only one large mix of amalgam is used then the later portions of the material will have begun to set before they are condensed into the cavity and this will lead to a deterioration in the properties of the restoration.

Mechanical condensation

This is normally carried out using a vibrating instrument. A variety of handpieces and handpiece attachments are available which provide this vibration. The actual vibration is transmitted to the amalgam by means of a series of condenser points of varying shapes and sizes to provide access to the different types of cavity (Fig. 7.11). The simpler types of vibrator provide condensation only in an axial direction, but the better types of vibrator, such as the Bergendal amalgam vibrator, provide both axial and lateral condensation for the filling material.

A small increment of amalgam is placed in the cavity from an amalgam carrier and vibrated using the largest condenser point that will conveniently fit within the cavity. This initial increment

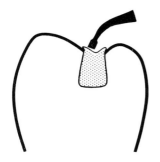

Fig. 7.12 Shaping the excess amalgam during condensation aids subsequent carving.

is condensed across the floor of the cavity and firmly into the appropriate line angles. A further increment is added and this process is repeated. As the cavity is filled, mercury-rich amalgam will accumulate on the surface of the packed material. This should be removed with an excavator and the incremental filling and condensing continued until the amalgam fills the cavity and lies in excess over the margins of the restoration. The surface of the restoration is finally condensed with one of the specially shaped points which will tend to form the contour of the filling to harmonise with that of the contour of the tooth.

Summary

There are two prerequisites for the preparation of strong amalgam. One is the close approximation of the particles of the filling material and the other is the reduction of the mercury content to a satisfactory level. If spherical alloys are used, even with an alloy:mercury ratio of more than 1:1, it will be found during condensation and carving that the amalgam feels softer and more plastic than with conventional alloys. This does not indicate an abnormally high residual mercury content but is a characteristic feature of the material.

Some types of amalgam set more rapidly and greater speed is then required in condensing and carving.

MATRICES

Where a cavity has a substantial part of one wall missing it is essential that some form of replacement for this wall is provided if amalgam is to be condensed satisfactorily into the cavity. The replacement for such a missing wall is known as a matrix. The essential functions of such a matrix are:

- To retain the amalgam in the cavity during condensation.
- To withstand the pressures involved so that adequate condensation of the amalgam can be produced.
- To ensure good adaptation of the restoration to the margins of the approximal box and to avoid excess amalgam gingivally.
- To ensure the restoration of the contact area and the external contour of the approximal surface of the tooth.

In addition the matrix should:

- Be easy to apply and remove.
- Not traumatise the tissues.
- Not react with the filling materials.

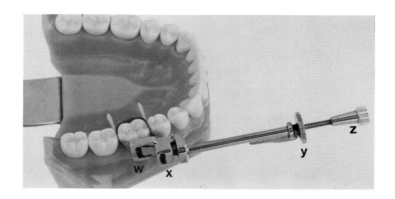

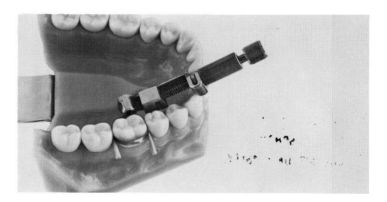

Fig. 7.13 (*Upper*) Bonnalie matrix.
Note slot *w* where band passes through
the head of the retainer; clamp *x* which
secures the ends of the band; knob *y*
which moves clamp *x* backwards and
forwards in relation to slot *w*; knob *z*
which tightens clamp *x* on to the band;
wedges at the gingival of the matrix
band. (*Lower*) Tofflemire matrix. Note
that because of its angled shaft this
retainer can be placed either lingually
or buccally; wedges at the gingival of
the matrix band.

A matrix for an amalgam cavity is manufactured of metal as
other materials are not strong enough to withstand the pressures of
condensation. It usually consists of a metal band completely
encircling the tooth held at one side by a clamp and wedged against
the gingival margin of the tooth approximately.

Pre-shaped wooden wedges are available. If it is not to produce

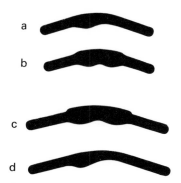

Fig. 7.14 Matrix bands. Arcuate bands for Bonnalie, Tofflemire or Nyström matrices: (*a*) premolar MO or DO, (*b*) premolar MOD, (*c*) molar MOD, (*d*) molar MO or DO.

a deficient contact, a wedge must always be placed well clear of the contact area, but when correctly positioned against the gingival margin it serves two functions. One is to adapt the matrix to the margin of the cavity and the other is to produce a very slight separation of the teeth. Good adaptation avoids gingival excess on the restoration and the slight separation ensures that when the wedge and the band are removed the approximal surfaces will come into contact taking up the space left by the removal of the matrix band.

Commonly used matrices are the Bonnalie, Tofflemire, Nyström, Siqveland and Automatrix.

Bonnalie

This matrix retainer (Fig. 7.13) uses arcuate bands (Fig. 7.14). The band passes completely around the tooth and through slot *w* in the shaft of the retainer. The ends of the band are held on the buccal side by the simple clamp mechanism *x*. Knob *z* is used to tighten clamp *x* on to the matrix band whilst knob *y* is used to move clamp *x* backwards and forwards along the shaft of the matrix retainer, thus increasing or decreasing the length of band available to pass around the tooth. These bands have projections along one margin which can be arranged to correspond with the approximal box or boxes of the cavity. Arcuate bands are shorter along the smaller arc (lower borders in Fig. 7.14) than along the larger arc (upper borders in Fig. 7.14), and when curved to pass around the tooth produce a smaller diameter circle at the gingival than at the occlusal. This, plus the gingival projections, ensures some degree of gingival adaptation. Contouring of the band with pliers and the use of wedges are, however, still indicated.

Tofflemire

This matrix employs the same principles as the Bonnalie but the retainer is angled (Fig. 7.13) instead of straight. This ensures that it is less likely to be displaced by the lip and because of the angulation of the shaft of the retainer it can also be placed on the lingual aspect of the tooth. This allows a continuous strip of band to pass around the buccal surface of the tooth and is occasionally useful in the packing of large buccal extensions.

Nyström

The Nyström matrix also uses arcuate bands but employs a pair of

Fig. 7.15 (*Upper*) Siqveland matrix, (*lower*) Nyström matrix. Compare swivel arm *w* with angled slots *x*, and the complex clamps *yy* with the simple clamp *z*.

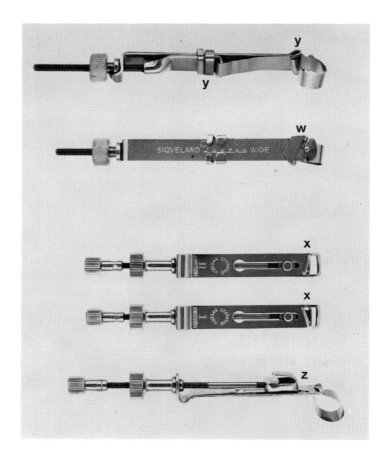

matrix retainers with inclined slots (Fig. 7.15); one for the upper left and lower right and one for the upper right and lower left. Provided that the correct retainer is selected the sloping groove will accentuate the gingival constriction as the matrix is tightened around the tooth. This improves gingival adaptation but does not eliminate the necessity for contouring and wedging.

Siqveland

This matrix does not use arcuate bands. It employs a simple strip matrix band and gains its gingival adaptation from one end of this band being attached to a swivelling arm (Fig. 7.15). As the band is placed and tightened the swivelling arm engages in the notch at the gingival border of the shaft of the retainer. The arm then swivels

Fig. 7.16 Caulk Automatrix, with Automate (*above*) which is inserted into the Autolock (*below*) and used to tighten the matrix band around the tooth. After use the Autolock loop is cut off and the band removed.

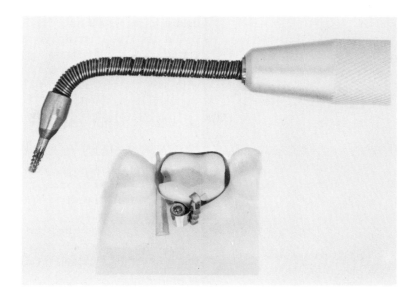

so as to produce a longer effective working length at the occlusal border of the band than at the gingival. The adaptation of this matrix to the gingival margin of the approximal box is good but as the bands have no gingival protections to correspond with the approximal boxes it is necessary to seat the matrix over the crown of the tooth until the gingival margin of the band has passed the gingival margins of these boxes. This may result in trauma to the buccal and lingual gingivae or, when filling an MO or DO, to the interdental papilla of the unaffected approximal area. It is possible to contour the band but this is time consuming, as is re-threading a new band. Despite these disadvantages the firm grip of this matrix around the gingival area makes it extremely stable and it is very useful in cases where the loss of tooth substance has been extensive.

Automatrix

This consists of an arcuate band coiled round to form a ring matrix (Fig. 7.16). Each ring is fitted with its own locking device (Autolock loop, Fig. 7.16a). They are available in several widths and a tool (Automate) is provided to tighten the matrix. The band is placed around the tooth with the Autolock loop in the centre of the buccal or lingual surface. The gingival contour is checked and alterations may be made by removing the band and adjusting with crown shears, rotating stones or contouring pliers. The matrix is held in place with a finger and the strip tightened by rotating the end of the Automate in the small coil (Fig. 7.16a). Wedges are placed and the amalgam packed and carved. The matrix is removed by clipping off the projecting end of the Autolock loop with wire cutters and then sliding the band away from the tooth.

CARVING AND POLISHING

In carving and polishing amalgam restorations the objectives are:

- To remove excess mercury-rich amalgam.
- To remove excess amalgam at the margins of the restorations.
- To ensure that the restoration is in harmony with the patient's occlusion.
- To produce modified but distinct anatomical contour, particularly of the marginal ridge.
- To produce a smooth polished surface to the restoration.

The first four objectives are best achieved at the stage of carving. It must be remembered that immediately after packing, the amalgam is readily amenable to shaping and removal. Once set this is infinitely more time consuming.

When the packing is complete and the material has started to set it should be carefully carved using a sharp instrument such as a Ward's or a Hollenbach carver or a probe. The smaller the restoration the smaller is the carver required. These instruments should be used to scrape or cut the amalgam and they should move along the margin of the cavity in such a way that they tend to force amalgam towards the margin of the tooth rather than away from it. In doing this the outer layer of mercury-rich amalgam should be removed. Finally, the surface may be smoothed by gentle rubbing or burnishing with a rounded condenser.

After 24 hours or more the restoration may be trimmed and polished. Any remaining marginal excess is removed and the surface is brought to a smooth shiny state through the gentle use of finishing burs. If carving has been carried out correctly the amount of trimming required is minimal but where positive 'catches' remain or inappropriate contours are found these must be removed or corrected. Once smooth and shiny the restoration may be polished using either bristle brushes or rubber cups, in conjunction with pumice and whiting or zinc oxide. A thick paste of pumice and glycerine (or water) is first applied to eliminate any remaining minor irregularities. The area is syringed with air and water spray and then dried. Whiting or zinc oxide, either dry or with a small amount of alcohol, is then used to obtain a high polish.

Two points should be noted:

- Polishing, particularly with dry agents, must be carried out carefully as it is easy to overheat the amalgam.
- The contours of the restoration must be guarded with care as over-enthusiastic polishing can eliminate valuable features.

Placing and finishing of the restoration

In all cases prior to the placing of an amalgam restoration, the cavity must be cleaned, dried and isolated from moisture contamination. Non gamma 2 alloys now appear to be the materials of choice. Those currently available contain a large proportion of spherical particles, therefore hand condensation techniques are described throughout.

CLASS I

A small increment of amalgam is placed in the base of the cavity using an amalgam carrier and is then packed firmly into place using a small amalgam condenser. The amalgam is condensed axially on to the floor of the cavity and laterally into the line angles. When this initial increment is firmly condensed in the cavity a further one is added and the procedure continued. The areas on which the condenser presses must overlap so that no amalgam escapes thorough condensation. It is essential to condense the amalgam throughout if a strong restoration is to be produced. It is not sufficient merely to pack the amalgam loosely in the deeper parts of the cavity and then condense the surface layers thoroughly. As incremental addition and packing is continued a quantity of softer amalgam will occur on the surface of the restoration, and this must be removed. As the final increments are placed, the surface of the amalgam is packed to approximate to the contour of the tooth (Fig. 7.12).

The restoration is carved using a carver held so that the blade is at right angles to the margin of the cavity and the tip positioned along the line which the central fissure system of the tooth should follow (Fig. 7.17). By gently scraping this blade back and forth it is possible to remove amalgam so as to reproduce the normal fissure system of the tooth. The objective is not to reproduce the fissure system precisely but to provide a modified rather more gentle contour which will be more easily cleaned.

If the depth of the occlusal fissures can be reduced slightly, a stronger edge can be provided for the restoration (Fig. 7.18).

When carving is complete the patient is asked to 'Gently close

Fig. 7.17 Ward's carver in position for occlusal carving.

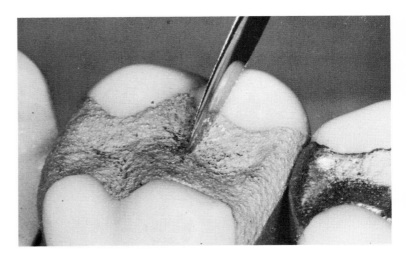

together' to check the occlusion. The surface of the restoration is examined for small marks made by the opposing teeth and if these are present the occlusal contour is modified to accommodate the opposing cusp. When no further marks are noted the patient is dismissed with a warning to avoid using the tooth for several hours.

At least 24 hours after the amalgam has been packed it may be trimmed with finishing burs and then polished. This is best carried out with a flame finishing bur held in the same way as the blade of the carver. The bur is rotated at 3000 r.p.m. and is passed gently over the surface of the tooth until a smooth, shiny scratch-free finish is produced. If scratches have to be eliminated from the depths of the fissure system then a small round or pear finishing bur should be used.

The amalgam is polished using the abrasives previously described on a rubber cup or bristle brush. The brushes and cups are rotated at 3000 r.p.m. and must be angled in such a manner that they maintain the contours of the restoration.

CLASS I WITH EXTENSION

This is treated in essentially the same manner as a simple Class I restoration. Some support, however, will have to be provided for the amalgam which is being packed into the extension if it is not to be displaced through the open side of the cavity. Where the extension is large this may be provided by fitting a matrix retainer and band on the tooth, but where the extension is small adequate support can be provided by placing a cellulose acetate strip against

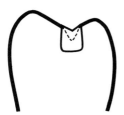

Fig. 7.18 Rounding of the fissure form of a restoration increases the bulk of the amalgam at the cavity margins.

the extension of the cavity and supporting this with a finger during the packing stage. A small excess of amalgam will be condensed out of the extension due to the soft texture of the finger supporting the strip but this can subsequently be burnished with a round-ended condenser. Carving and finishing are carried out in the same manner as for a simple Class I restoration.

CLASS II

A suitable matrix is placed in position on the tooth and firmly wedged gingivally. The first increments of amalgam are placed into the buccal and lingual line angles of the approximal box and condensed firmly in both lateral and axial directions using a small cylindrical condenser. The whole of the gingival floor of the approximal box is covered and thoroughly condensed. The box is then incrementally filled and condensed until it is level with the pulpal floor of the occlusal portion of the cavity. Care must be taken to ensure that the amalgam is condensed very firmly up to the buccal and lingual cavo-surface angles. At this stage the occlusal portion of the cavity is treated in essentially the same manner as a Class I restoration but continuing right along the occlusal surface up to and including the approximal box and packing the material hard against the matrix band and out towards the buccal and lingual cavo-surface angles. The whole cavity is packed to excess, as for the Class I restoration.

The parts of the occlusal surface directly related to the cusps are contoured with a carver as in a Class I restoration, but the approximal area requires special treatment. The marginal ridge is carefully reproduced at the margin of the tooth closely related to the matrix band using a carver or a probe. The position of a natural marginal ridge on a comparable tooth should be noted in order to assist the inexperienced student in placing the marginal ridge in the correct position. The triangular grooves immediately within the marginal ridge must be clearly reproduced if a satisfactory occlusion is to be provided, the correct paths of food shedding produced, and impaction of food between the approximal surfaces of the teeth avoided.

By this stage the amalgam will be partially set and it is safe to release the matrix retainer, remove the wedges and gently ease out the matrix band from between the restoration and the adjacent tooth. This can best be done by using a gentle bucco-lingual motion on the band so that it slides backwards and forwards at the same time as it is worked towards the occlusal surface of the tooth. Where the retainer can be removed separately, this should be done to facilitate the safe removal of the band. Immediately the matrix band has been removed the gingival margin of the restoration is checked for excess amalgam with a probe. Any excess is removed and then similar treatment is given to the buccal and lingual margins of the approximal box. At this stage the patient is asked to 'Gently close together', to check the occlusion. Any excess force on the amalgam at this stage may well lead to fracture of the restoration. When the occlusion is correct and all loose amalgam is removed interdentally the patient is dismissed with a warning not to use the tooth for several hours.

Trimming is once again carried out using a flame finishing bur on the occlusal surface and passing the same bur into the embrasures from the buccal and lingual sides of the tooth will trim any excess in this region. The occlusal surface and the accessible portions of the approximal surfaces are polished using bristle brushes or rubber cups and the conventional abrasives. The gingival area of the restoration may be gently polished using linen, sandpaper or cuttle strips passed gingival to the contact area. They are passed gently to and fro along the gingival margin of the restoration and provide a reasonably smooth surface in this area. If a gross excess of amalgam is found in this area, then usually the only satisfactory method of dealing with it is to remove the restoration and start again. It is not desirable to polish the contact area of the restoration as any removal of material in this area will tend to lead to a deficient contact with resultant food packing and trauma to the interdental papilla. A completed fully extended restoration is shown in Fig. 7.19.

CLASS V

This cavity is packed in essentially the same manner as a Class I restoration and is filled to slight excess. The restoration is carved using a carver or a probe, held at right angles to the cavity margins. Care must be taken to maintain the convexity of the restoration and to ensure that no excess material is left at the gingival margin. The buccal contour of the restoration should be slightly exaggerated at this stage as trimming and polishing of the restoration will lead to a reduction in this convexity.

The trimming of the restoration is once again carried out with flame finishing burs but extreme care must be taken to avoid traumatising the gingival tissues. Polishing is carried out with cups or brushes and the usual abrasives. The convexity of the restoration must not be eliminated. An extensive restoration is shown in Fig. 7.19.

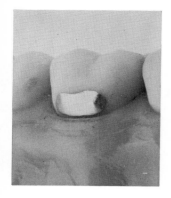

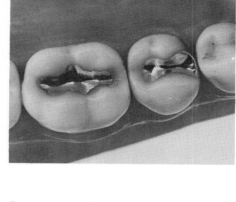

Fig. 7.19 Finished amalgam restorations: (*left*) Class V, (*right*) Class II MO and Class I.

Larger amalgam restorations

Where the spread of caries is very extensive, more complex amalgam restorations may be required than the basic ones so far described. These may be used as completed restorations or they may form the foundations for gold veneer crowns. Two larger types will be described, firstly, cusp replacement with pin retention used where caries has completely undermined one or more cusps and, secondly, which Class II and Class V cavities extend into one another.

CUSP REPLACEMENT

If whole cusps have been undermined it may still be possible to restore a tooth with amalgam by removing the whole of the affected cusp and replacing it with amalgam (Fig. 7.20). This apparently drastic treatment is necessary in order to ensure an adequate bulk of amalgam to withstand the heavy occlusal stresses.

Retention for these restorations is provided by the use of self-threading pins placed within the dentine. Different diameters of pin are available ranging from 0.8 to 0.5 mm in diameter. These pins must avoid the enamel–dentine junction and the pulp. They must penetrate 2–3 mm into the dentine and project about 2–3 mm into the amalgam restoration if satisfactory retention is to be provided. The threads on self-threading pins provide adequate retention, both for the pin within the tooth and for the amalgam around the pin, but pins may be inserted at a slight angle to the axis of the tooth and to each other, or bent slightly, in order to increase their retentive effect. Care must be taken to ensure that there is

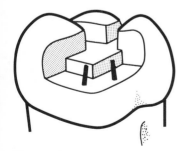

Fig. 7.20 MOD amalgam cavity for replacement of one cusp. Two small self-threading pins are shown in position.

Fig. 7.21 (*left to right*) Twist drill, self-shearing pin with latch type shank, self-shearing pin with tapered latch type self-centring shank, pin with plastic latch type shank and chuck for insertion by hand.

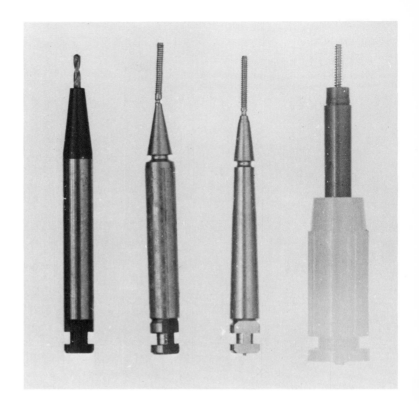

good access to all sides of the pins so that amalgam can be thoroughly condensed around them.

The simplest form of this type of cavity will be described, that is an MOD in a molar from which one cusp has been lost.

Preparation

The basic MOD cavity is prepared as described previously. The whole of the affected cusp is removed until a sound floor is established for the cavity. The precise form of this will vary considerably from case to case depending on the distribution of the caries, but one example is shown in Fig. 7.20. Pinholes are then sunk well away from the enamel–dentine junction, the estimated position of the pulp and the bifurcation or trifurcation of the roots. Small 'marker' holes are made with a No. $\frac{1}{2}$ round bur at the appropriate sites. A twist drill (Fig. 7.21) revolving at not more than 800 r.p.m. is used to produce the 2–3 mm deep holes and self-threading pins are screwed in using a hand chuck or a

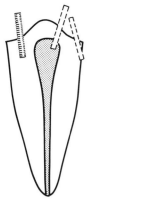

Fig. 7.22 Pins must be correctly angled to stay within the dentine.

low-speed handpiece (Fig. 7.21). In the latter case either the pin assembly or the handpiece must contain a torque limiting device.

Where more than one cusp is missing up to two pins per half premolar and three pins per half molar are inserted. Complete amalgam cores can be retained by between four and six pins. With very large cavities it is difficult to find safe areas in which to place pins. Great care must be taken to assess the external shape of the tooth and the positions of the bifurcation or trifurcation, the pulp chamber and the pulp horns. The latter two will vary with the age of the patient and the history of the tooth. As well as the choice of site the angle at which the pin is sunk can also be critical (Fig. 7.22).

Lining

A base is placed in the normal manner except that great care must be taken to avoid reducing the effective length of pin available to retain the amalgam.

Placing the filling

Where only one cusp is to be replaced a normal matrix can be used and the cavity is filled in the usual manner. Particular care is taken to condense amalgam thoroughly around the pins and the finished restoration is carved. Once the basic occlusal anatomy has been produced, the matrix band is carefully removed and the final carving of the approximal and buccal contours completed. It is of vital importance to ensure that no abnormal occlusal stress is placed on the newly constructed amalgam cusp during the 24 hours following condensation. The occlusion of the cusp must be checked with great care and the patient warned not to eat hard foods in that area. After this period the restoration can be trimmed and polished in the usual manner.

The loss of more than one cusp in a molar, or of only one in a premolar, frequently leads to difficulty in retaining a normal matrix on the tooth during condensation of the amalgam. In view of this and the relative weakness of the newly packed amalgam it is advisable in these cases either to use an Automatrix or to contour a copper ring to fit around the tooth. This ring can then be used as a matrix and the amalgam condensed within it. A ring of suitable diameter is selected and one end cut with crown shears to match the gingival contour of the preparation. The edge is smoothed with a rotary abrasive and the ring tried in position. It should fit

tightly around the neck of the tooth and the margin should extend
1 mm past the margin of the preparation. If the fit and contour are
essentially satisfactory, minor adjustments can be made with a
rotary abrasive and contouring pliers. The occlusal margin is then
cut to be clear of the occlusion and similarly smoothed. The ring is
finally positioned on the tooth, wedged approximally and amalgam condensed within it. It can be left in position for 24 hours
after condensation helping to protect the set amalgam, but if it is
left longer than this it will lead to gingival inflammation.
Alternatively, it may be cut with a bur, used at high speed, and
removed at the same visit. This ring technique tends to produce an
inadequately shaped amalgam restoration with deficient contact
areas and is most commonly used when constructing amalgam
cores for gold veneer crowns (Chapter 9).

CONFLUENT CLASS II AND CLASS V RESTORATIONS

Where caries on the buccal or lingual surface of a tooth connects
with caries on the approximal surface a potentially difficult
situation results. The caries can be removed and the cavity
prepared relatively easily using the techniques described for Class
II and Class V cavity preparations. The shape of the resulting
cavity, however, makes it impossible to condense amalgam
satisfactorily into both sections simultaneously. This problem is
overcome by filling the Class V part with a quick-setting
temporary filling material and packing the Class II cavity in the
normal manner. At a subsequent visit the temporary dressing is
removed from the Class V section and the amalgam wall of this
cavity trimmed with a bur to produce a clean surface and some
degree of undercut. This cavity can then be packed with amalgam
in the usual manner.

This principle can be applied on either the buccal or the lingual
side of the tooth on one or both ends of the Class V cavity.

Replacement and repair of amalgam restorations

When replacing a restoration it is important to remove the old
filling without increasing the size of the cavity, unless this is
required for some reason such as the removal of caries. The
instrument of choice is usually a small diamond fissure bur in the
high-speed handpiece. Cuts must be made within the amalgam
allowing segments of the filling to be removed with an excavator
and leaving the cavity walls untouched. After any necessary
modifications to the cavity the unaltered sections of cavity wall

should be finished with a Baker-Curson bur and the cavity lined and filled.

In view of the work of Elderton (1977), when a large restoration is essentially sound except for one obvious defect, consideration should be given to repairing that defect rather than replacing the whole restoration. This procedure is even more relevant to pin-retained restorations. In a severely damaged tooth the amount of dentine suitable for receiving pins is small and when the tooth is first restored the best sites for the pins are chosen. These pins are inevitably lost when the filling is removed and the replacement of a multi-pin restoration can prove difficult. A careful repair can often provide a safe, simple and satisfactory alternative. The filling material and any demineralised tooth tissue around the defect is removed with a bur at low speed until it can be clearly seen that the remaining restoration and tooth tissue are sound. The tooth is then examined to ensure that the rest of the filling is completely stable and that the new cavity is retentive. The margins of the cavity are finished and a lining and filling placed.

References

ELDERTON R.J. (1977) *Assessment of the Quality of Dental Care*. Ed. H. Allred. pp. 45–81. London Hospital Medical College.
LUFKIN A.W. (1948) *A History of Dentistry*, 2nd edn., p. 272. Kimpton, London.
RODDA J.C (1972) *N.Z. dent. J.* **68**, 132–138.

Chapter 8
Aesthetic restorations

When restoring carious cavities in the anterior teeth it is important that the restorative material should simulate as closely as possible the natural tooth substance which it replaces because these teeth will be visible during normal functional movements of the lips. However, the development of an ideal aesthetic restorative material has proved difficult and the current materials are still not completely satisfactory. This book stresses the need for prevention of dental caries and the difficulties in developing good aesthetic materials reinforce the desirability of preventing caries, particularly in anterior teeth. The majority of patients who attend for regular dental care are concerned about the appearance of their teeth and this should be used to increase their motivation towards prevention.

For many years silicate cement was the main aesthetic filling material, it was based on a combination of phosphoric acid and alumino-silicate glass powder. Initial appearance was good but it stained readily. It had a low compressive and tensile strength and did not bond directly to tooth substance. Autopolymerising acrylic resin filling materials became commercially available about 1945 but proved unsatisfactory due to low abrasion resistance, poor colour stability and a high coefficient of thermal expansion compared to tooth tissue.

The materials currently in use are the composite and glass ionomer cements. Composite cements became available in the late 1960s. They consist of a resin matrix and an organic filler. The filler reduces the thermal expansion and increases the abrasion resistance of the material. The resin used in most composites is based on the reaction product of bisphenol A and glycidyl methacrylate.

The inorganic fillers used include aluminium silicate compounds and glass spheres and rods. A potential weakness in these materials is the bond between the filler and the matrix which allows the relatively large particles of filler to be dislodged so that an abraded surface is always rough. More recently, much finer filler particles have been used in the microfine composites and with these a high surface finish can be developed by grinding and polishing. This finish is currently thought to be relatively resistant to further abrasion (Wilson, Davies & von Frauenhofer 1981).

Composites can be retained in the cavity either by conventional mechanical retention within the dentine or by the micro-mechanical bond of resin tags within the enamel, if this has been etched with an acid. Variations in the effect of etching and the physical structure of the bond are well discussed by Crawford & Whittaker (1977). The ability of acid-etched composite to bond to enamel has been used to:

- Splint mobile teeth.
- Retain Rochette bridges or orthodontic brackets.
- Modify tooth contours to aid retention of dentures.
- Improve the appearance of mis-shaped or intrinsically stained teeth.

The glass ionomer cements are based on the reaction between an alumino-silicate glass and polycarboxylic acids, mainly polyacrylic acid. This results in a cored structure of incompletely reacted particles of the glass bound together by a metal-polyacrylate gel matrix. These cements bond specifically to enamel and dentine; they are tooth coloured but currently lack true translucency.

The aim of much current research is the development of a truly aesthetic strong and stable filling material which will adhere to enamel and dentine whilst being non-irritant to the pulp. Considerable progress has been made in recent years and in some circumstances the mechanical aspects of traditional cavity design have become less important. As materials develop, cavity preparation and other techniques will change so this chapter must be read in association with recent research reports and the manufacturer's instructions for specific materials.

Principles of cavity design for anterior aesthetic restorations

The essential features of the physical characteristics of the aesthetic restorative materials which affect the design of these cavities are:

- The material when mixed is plastic and subsequently hardens. It can, therefore, be placed into cavities in which undercuts provide positive mechanical retention.
- All areas on anterior teeth should be readily cleansable by the careful patient, and some cements slowly release fluoride, so minimal extension is the norm.

- The tensile and compressive strengths and the abrasion resistance of these materials are much lower than those of dental enamel. In the preparation of cavities for these materials only the minimum amount of tooth surface should be removed.
- A tooth contains many subtle variations in colour across its surface. The restorative materials are essentially simple in colour and so far all tend to stain and discolour with time. Only the minimum area of restorative material should be visible on the labial surface of the tooth.
- Aesthetic materials are potentially irritant to the pulp, so a lining is usually required.

CLASS I AND CLASS II

The compressive and tensile strength of aesthetic materials would normally be considered inadequate for cavities of this type. It has been suggested that some of them may be used cautiously in minimal cavities where special circumstances exist. Small mesial lesions on premolars may sometimes be restored using a technique similar to that described for labial approach Class III cavities.

CLASS III

Caries related to the contact area of an anterior tooth must normally be approached through either the labial or lingual surface of the tooth, the direction of approach being determined by the position of the carious lesion. Where access is available equally from either direction the lingual approach is usually the one of choice in upper anterior teeth as the subsequent restoration will show least from the labial surface. If incisors are imbricated (Fig. 8.1) one cavity may be prepared from the lingual and one from the labial. In lower incisors where appearance is less important and access to the lingual surface of the teeth is more difficult, the labial approach is the one of choice.

The size of the lesion will influence both the form of cavity and the filling materials used. Where appearance is at a premium composite should be selected. If a cavity can be kept small best aesthetics are achieved using traditional mechanical retention but in larger cavities, where it is difficult or impossible to produce an incisal retention pit, an acid-etch technique should be used. When appearance is less critical small cavities may be filled with glass ionomer cement. Mechanical retention is less important with this material and it has a useful fluoride leaching effect. Lingual and labial approach Class III cavities may appear very different but

Fig. 8.1 Imbricated central and lateral incisors.

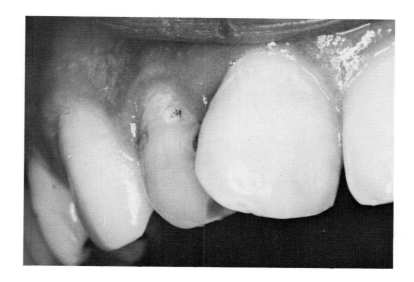

they have much in common. This is best illustrated by considering first the cavity which can be prepared where there is a space in the arch and where the approximal surface of the tooth can be approached directly.

Direct approach (adjacent tooth removed)

Access and removal of caries is carried out with a round bur in a conventional handpiece. When the caries has been removed the outline of the cavity will generally be triangular conforming approximately to the shape of the pre-existing contact area and related carious lesion (Fig. 8.2).

Mechanical form in this cavity is essentially that of a simple flat-floored cavity with the retention being provided by an incisal pit and a gingival groove. These are positioned as shown in Fig. 8.2 (*left*) and are produced with a small round bur in the conventional handpiece. In the majority of cavities it is not possible to place labial and lingual retention grooves. The labio-lingual curvature of the tooth would result in unsupported enamel margins if such grooves were prepared. The cavity margins are trimmed with a chisel or a Baker-Curson bur until the enamel margin is moderately strong and the cavo-surface angle is a right angle. Compromise may be necessary since removal of all unsupported enamel may leave the cavity without adequate retention and more filling material may be visible.

123 *Aesthetic restorations*

Fig. 8.2 Class III cavities.
(*Left*) direct approach; (*centre*) labial
approach; (*right*) lingual approach.

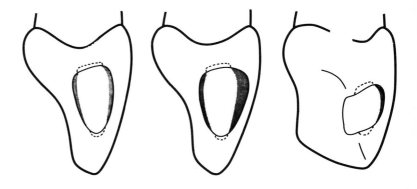

Biological form No specific modifications are made to the outline of this cavity, but if the cavity is not deep enough to accommodate both the liner and filling it must be deepened accordingly.

Labial approach

Access is gained from the approximo-labial aspect of the tooth using a round bur in a handpiece (Fig. 8.3). Care must be taken not to slip and damage the adjacent tooth. Where a sound layer of enamel covers the caries it may be desirable to make an entry into the carious lesion using a small round bur in the air turbine. It must be stressed that only the minimal amount of sound tooth substance should be removed and high-speed instruments are frequently not required.

Removal of caries and the production of *Mechanical and Biological form* are carried out in essentially the same way as for a direct approach cavity. The lingual margin of the cavity should be positioned just clear of the contact area to allow a matrix to pass between the teeth, and the finished cavity should appear similar to the direct approach cavity except that the labial wall is flared sufficiently to allow access and vision from the labial surface (Fig. 8.2, *centre*). The contour of the labial margin of the cavity must be treated with great care. Wherever possible it should have a gentle curve which harmonises with the natural contours of the tooth so that even if the restoration subsequently discolours the appearance will not be unduly offensive. If, due to careless cutting, the visual continuity of the tooth has been broken then a stained restoration is much more noticeable.

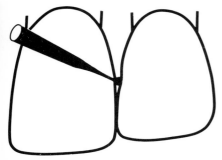

Fig. 8.3 Small round bur approaching the approximo-labial aspect of the upper lateral incisor.

Lingual approach

Access is gained through the lingual surface of the tooth and, as the contour of the lingual margin of the cavity does not influence the appearance of the restoration, a rather square outline may be produced, providing good vision and access to all parts of the cavity (Fig. 8.2, *right*).

Mechanical form   Retention against mesio-distal and bucco-lingual displacement is provided by a carefully placed incisal pit and gingival groove and the enamel margins should be trimmed to remove weak enamel.

Biological form   The precise position of the labial margins of these cavities should be carefully assessed. The object of the lingual approach is to avoid the restoration being easily visible so, unless caries extends on to the labial surface, the labial margin of the cavity should be positioned so that it is just possible to pass a matrix strip between the teeth. The cavity must also be deep enough to accommodate both liner and filling.

Preparation   The round end of a dome-ended fissure bur is used to gain access through the lingual surface. Where the enamel is intact an air turbine should be used for a few seconds to penetrate the enamel. If the caries extends on to the lingual surface conventional speeds are adequate and much of the caries can be removed using the one bur. Where adequate access and vision cannot be gained through the initial entry, the outline of the access cavity is modified by moving the bur incisally or gingivally until adequate access is obtained.

A final check is made with an excavator to ensure that all caries has been removed. An incisal pit and a gingival groove are prepared with a small round bur to provide positive retention. The incisal and gingival margins of the cavity are planed with a hatchet chisel to remove weak enamel and the labial margin is planed with a margin trimmer. Final trimming of the lingual margin is carried out with a Baker-Curson bur.

Summary

The essential features of a small Class III cavity for use with an aesthetic restorative material are:

● The surface area of the cavity should be kept as small as is compatible with satisfactory access and visibility.

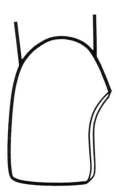

Fig. 8.4 Labial view of cavity for a Class IV acid-etch composite restoration.

● There should be minimal interference with the labial surface of the tooth. Where labial involvement is essential the outline of the cavity should harmonise with the tooth contours.
● There must always be sufficient depth in the cavity to accommodate a lining as well as a filling.
● Adequate pit and groove retention must be provided unless a bonding technique is being used.

Larger cavities

Caries sometimes extends so far incisally that to create a retention pit would weaken the incisal edge. It is possible to provide retention for such a Class III restoration by using an acid-etch technique.

Access and removal of caries   This is carried out from the lingual side as in the smaller Class III cavities but access is simplified by the greater amount of tooth tissue which has been softened or destroyed, and it is this which will largely control the outline of the cavity.

Mechanical form   Retention pits and grooves may be used to supplement the acid-etch retention where this is practicable. When the gingival margin of the cavity is in cementum a gingival groove must be developed in the dentine as the composite will not bond on to this margin. All enamel margins should be given a half-thickness 135° bevel with a fine carrot-shaped diamond at low speed and then finished with a flame-shaped Baker-Curson bur at high speed.

CLASS IV

Composite materials are not ideal for restoring Class IV cavities because of their low abrasion resistance. However, a cavity involving the incisal edge can be restored using a composite cement with an acid-etch technique.

Preparation   All caries and unsupported enamel are removed from the tooth and a half-thickness 135° bevel cut on all enamel margins. This completes the preparation (Fig. 8.4).

CLASS V

The principles underlying the design of Class V cavities for use

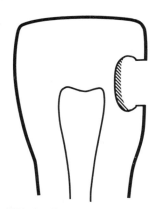

Fig. 8.5 Cross-section of an incisor tooth showing the lining of a Class III cavity. Note that the lining covers the area of the cavity floor from which tubules run to the pulp.

with aesthetic restorative materials are identical to those for amalgam cavities, as is the technique of preparation. Where it is difficult to obtain mechanical retention for extensive restorations the enamel margins may be bevelled and acid-etch composite placed. Where appearance is less critical glass ionomer cements in unbevelled cavities may be used.

Taking a shade

The aesthetic restorative materials are available in a range of shades and care must be taken in selecting the most appropriate shade for a particular tooth. The tooth should be clean and the shade taken before it is isolated, as superficial staining, abnormal dehydration and the colour of an adjacent rubber dam may all affect the apparent colour of the tooth. The manufacturer's shade guide usually consists of a number of tooth-shaped colour samples. These are compared to the surface of the tooth and the appropriate colour is chosen. With some materials it is possible to mix the base materials of two shades to provide intermediate ones, whilst with other materials special modifier colours are available to enable detailed variations in shade to be reproduced. It may be found useful to take the shade whilst waiting for the local anaesthetic to take effect.

Cavity isolation

All cavities in which aesthetic restorative materials are to be placed must be kept free of moisture whilst the material is being inserted and setting. Water interferes with the setting reactions of some of the materials, adversely affects the physical properties of the restoration and produces poor marginal adaptation. Contamination with blood pigments can alter the colour. The application of a rubber dam (Chapter 11) is the best possible method of isolation. It can be used to isolate almost all Class III as well as many Class V cavities. Where a cavity extends very far sub-gingivally it may not be possible to place a rubber dam. The area may then be isolated by using a saliva ejector and cotton wool roll in the labial sulcus.

Linings

COMPOSITE

The pulpal floor of the cavity should be covered with a thin layer of liner (Fig. 8.5) as described in Chapter 6. When using an acid-etch technique the liner should be placed before etching is carried out and its integrity should be checked after etching has taken place.

Although these materials are less irritant to the pulp than the composites, it is still good practice to apply a coating of liner to any newly cut dentine adjacent to the pulp. This will still leave the walls and part of the floor free for direct bonding with the cement. Again, the liner should be applied before acid conditioner is placed in the cavity.

Aesthetic restorative materials

COMPOSITE

The manipulation of this group of materials varies. They are presented in two basic forms, light activated and chemically activated.

With the light activated resins the constituent materials are mixed, applied to the tooth, held in place with a matrix and polymerised using an intense beam of light. These materials have the advantage of an unlimited working time which allows extended manipulation of the matrix, but unless great care is taken the depth of cure is unreliable.

Chemically activated resins have a limited working time and three types of systems are currently available:

● Two-dough systems: polymerisation occurs when the doughs are mixed together.
● Dough containing all ingredients except activator which is in a separate solution and is mixed with the dough before use.
● Powder–liquid system: the powder contains the inorganic filler and the activator, the liquid contains the monomer and any other components.

Mixing should be carried out in accordance with the manufacturer's instructions. When an acid-etch technique is to be used the enamel margins of the cavity are etched with a solution of phosphoric acid for approximately 1 minute. The agent is carefully washed away using an air-water spray for 10 seconds and the area thoroughly dried with a jet of oil-free air. The etched surface must then be kept untouched and scrupulously clean of any contamination.

These may be presented in pre-dispensed capsules for use in a mechanical mixer or as a powder and liquid to be mixed with a nichrome spatula on an agate slab. Correct proportioning and mixing is very important and the manufacturer's instructions should be followed with care. Before the filling is placed in the cavity this should be conditioned with a solution of citric acid for 20 seconds. The acid is then washed away and the area dried and maintained scrupulously clean as in an acid-etch composite technique.

Placing the restoration

CLASS III

Any preliminary etching or conditioning is carried out and the matrix prepared. This is a simple strip of cellulose acetate or one of the proprietary plastics. The matrix band is positioned approximally and a small wooden wedge placed at the gingival margin to adapt it to the tooth surface. Access can be gained to either a labial or a lingual approach cavity as shown in Fig. 8.6. If required, a layer of unfilled resin is flowed around the cavity margins, then a quantity of filling material is taken on a plastic-filling instrument, carefully inserted into the cavity and packed into the incisal and gingival areas. A second increment, judged to be *slightly* in excess of that required to fill the cavity, is then packed on to the first. The matrix band is drawn firmly around the tooth, the filling checked for good marginal adaptation and contour, and held firmly in position until the material is set. The filling material must be placed and the matrix positioned as rapidly as possible. The procedure must not take longer than 60 seconds with glass ionomer and chemically activated composite cements if the structure of the finished restoration is not to be disturbed. Once the initial set has occurred the matrix band is removed. This time is approximately 3 minutes after the insertion but the manufacturer's recommendations should be carefully followed. From this point cement and the composite materials require different treatment.

With the composite cements excess cannot easily be removed using hand instruments as the material is too hard. Rotary instruments should be used as little as possible to avoid disturbing the incompletely polymerised cement, but gingival or other troublesome excess should be removed with fine diamonds or

Fig. 8.6 Class III matrices. Cellulose acetate strip positioned and wedged for use with (*above*) labial approach cavity and (*below*) lingual approach cavity.

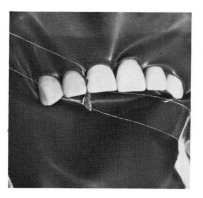

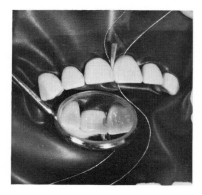

tungsten carbide finishing burs. Final trimming should be postponed to a later visit when polymerisation will be complete and the water content of the restoration will have become stabilised.

With glass ionomer cement any gross excess beyond the margins is removed using either a sharp excavator or scalpel and the restoration is immediately coated with copal ether varnish using tweezers and a pledget of cotton wool. This prevents the cement from losing or gaining water. Cutting instruments should be kept away from the margins of the restoration and care must be taken to direct these instruments so as to press the restoration against rather than away from the wall of the cavity. Fine trimming with stones at this stage would disturb and weaken the structure of the cement. Such trimming should be postponed until at least 24 hours after insertion unless there is lingual excess interfering with the occlusion, in which case it must be removed by stoning.

CLASS IV

These may be treated in the same way as Class III cavities, but nipping the incisal portion of the matrix band with two fingers to establish an incisal edge to the restoration. This technique provides good incisal adaptation but rather poor contour. Gross incisal excess can be readily trimmed with a diamond at high speed and, as newly mixed composite readily bonds to recently set uncontaminated material, additions can be made if required. Indeed, with large restorations an incremental approach may be deliberately adopted using either chemically activated or light activated resins. This simplifies the shaping of the filling and helps to ensure a consistent depth of cure.

Alternatively, a cellulose acetate crown form may be trimmed to just overlap the margin of the cavity. A small hole is made in the incisal edge so that the risk of air inclusion is reduced. The filled matrix is placed on the tooth and held in position until the material is set. Despite some excess material escaping through the incisal pin-hole there is a tendency for this technique to produce gingival excess which is very difficult to remove. Similar techniques using complete crown forms, custom-built silicone rubber matrices or free-hand incremental techniques can be used to restore whole crowns or build up peg-shaped laterals. With very extensive restorations it is difficult to produce an ideal gingival contour.

CLASS V

Metallic concave kidney-shaped matrices (Fig. 8.7) may be used which reproduce both the mesio-distal and inciso-gingival contours. They are soft enough to be swaged to produce good marginal apposition prior to mixing the cement. For ease of handling these matrices can be temporarily attached to a cylindrical condenser with varnish.

A slight excess of filling material is placed in the clean, dry cavity using a plastic-filling instrument. The matrix is positioned over it and held in position until the material is set. Light pressure only should be applied so that the matrix does not become distorted and the contour of the restoration lost. When the filling material has set, the matrix is removed and the restoration is then treated in the same way as described for Class III restorations.

Fig. 8.7 Class V matrices. (*Upper left*) different sizes of metallic concave matrices; (*upper right*) matrix attached to a cylindrical condenser with copal-ether varnish; (*lower left*) matrix placed in position on tooth; (*lower right*) matrix in position after filling has set prior to removal.

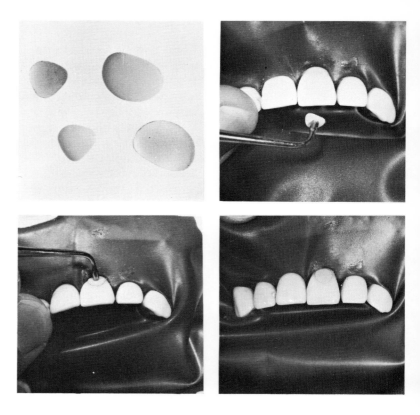

Finishing the restoration

With either cement no finishing is the best finishing. By this it is meant a perfectly adapted matrix leaving no excess at the margins will provide the best possible finish to the surface of the restoration. However, this ideal state of affairs frequently does not occur and some trimming of the restoration is necessary. Indeed, it has been suggested that trimming and polishing of microfine composites may be beneficial (Wilson *et al.* 1981). When finishing, the manufacturer's instructions should be carefully noted, diamond stones should be used for the removal of gross excess which is not near to the cavity margins; near the margins, and for final finishing, white abrasive stones are the instruments of choice. With the addition of flexible abrasive discs and strips this should provide an acceptable group for finishing these materials. The direction of rotation should always tend to force the restorative material against the wall of the cavity rather than pulling it away. Abrasive strips are used to trim the approximal gingival margin where this is necessary. The strip is passed through the interdental space and pulled carefully backwards and forwards against the excess cement. Trauma to the gingival tissues must be avoided. Petroleum jelly should be used as a lubricant when trimming glass ionomer cements. It should be noted that thin films of composite are extremely difficult to detect and very careful inspection of the finished restoration is required.

References

CRAWFORD P.J. & WHITTAKER D.K. (1977) *Brit. dent. J.* **143**, 261–266.
WILSON A.D. (1972) *National Bureau of Standards Special Publication* **354**, 85–92.
WILSON G.S., DAVIES E.H. & VON FRAUENHOFER J.A. (1981) *Brit. dent. J.* **151**, 335–338.

Chapter 9
Inlays and crowns

Some restorations are made directly in the mouth using rapid-setting materials which are mixed at the chairside, placed in the prepared cavity, and shaped in the mouth during and after setting. Examples of these are amalgam, composite and glass ionomer, all of which have been described earlier. The present chapter is concerned with restorations which are made wholly or partly in the laboratory; these include gold inlays, full veneer gold crowns, porcelain bonded to metal crowns and porcelain jacket crowns. The term veneer implies that the material is present in a comparatively thin layer on the surface of the tooth; a full veneer crown covers the whole of the natural crown while a partial veneer crown covers only part of it.

These *indirect* restorations can be divided into those which are mainly *intra-coronal*, that is enclosed within the crown, and those which are *extra-coronal*, and enclose the remaining natural crown of the tooth. The former are called *inlays* and the latter *crowns*, but the distinction between the two is not sharp; for example, full and partial veneer crowns may have intra-coronal extensions and inlays may have extra-coronal extensions. Most indirect restorations are made entirely in the laboratory on a replica of the prepared tooth, with its adjacent and opposing teeth, but some small inlays are first built up in wax in the mouth and then cast in gold in the laboratory.

Indirect restorations are sealed to the tooth with a rapid-setting cement. The currently available dental cements permit some marginal leakage (Grieve & Glyn Jones 1981) and do not exhibit true adhesion to both restoration and tooth; therefore the restorations must fit as accurately as possible along their margins so that the minimum of cement is exposed to the oral fluids. They must also fit accurately against all the internal walls to provide retention and stability. Tooth preparation for indirect restorations must be free from undercuts in one axis to allow the restoration to be seated (Fig. 9.1).

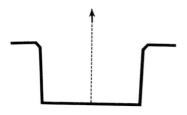

Fig. 9.1 Cross-section of a typical inlay cavity showing the flat floor, square internal angles, slightly divergent walls and bevelled cavo-surface angle. The dotted line represents the axis of withdrawal.

Indications for the use of inlays and crowns

Inlays are becoming less frequently used for simpler cavities and are generally reserved for those teeth where a special need exists, such as those weakened by caries and likely to fracture if not protected, or where retention is a problem. In both cases the ability to use a veneer covering part or all of the tooth surface enables a strong, durable restoration to be constructed. Crowns are used increasingly since it is now possible to cut tooth substance rapidly and because of the emergence of materials, such as porcelain bonded to metal, which give both strength and good appearance.

INLAYS

Class I

Inlays of this type are very rarely necessary but may be used as a matter of choice.

Class II

Inlays are rarely essential for small Class II cavities but may be used if desired. MOD inlays are indicated where tooth destruction has undermined and weakened cusps. If these cusps are not protected they may subsequently fracture leaving a difficult restorative problem. It is best to reduce the weak cusps and extend a veneer of metal over them thus spreading the load on to stronger areas.

Class III and Class IV

These inlays are not often indicated as the appearance of gold in anterior teeth is becoming less acceptable; composite restorations involve much less removal of tooth tissue and are simpler to make. Class III and Class IV inlays may occasionally be used as attachments for semi-fixed bridges.

Class V

Class V inlays make good restorations provided that they are aesthetically acceptable and that adequate retention is obtained. They can be used to aid the retention of partial dentures using ball-ended clasps. Retention for these inlays may be augmented by the use of pins; this design is particularly useful for the treatment of shallow cavities caused by abrasion or erosion. For complex cavities which extend around several cervical surfaces, direct restorations of amalgam, composite or glass ionomer materials are to be preferred.

CROWNS

These are used to restore teeth, parts of which have been extensively destroyed. They may also be used to retain bridges or accept rests or clasps of partial dentures.

Full veneer cast gold crowns

These are used only on molars or on premolars which are not important aesthetically. They can provide a strong, retentive restoration.

Partial veneer cast gold crowns

These are midway between MOD inlays and full veneer crowns and are indicated occasionally where buccal cusps are strong, lingual cusps weak, and additonal retention is needed.

Porcelain bonded to metal crowns

These give the valuable combination of good appearance and strength but are more expensive than gold or porcelain crowns and require more tooth destruction. Nevertheless, they are extensively used and form the basis of much bridge construction.

Porcelain jacket crowns

Made from aluminous porcelain, these are used almost entirely on incisor and canine teeth. They combine good appearance with adequate strength when used in sufficient thickness, but in thin section or under heavy load they may fracture. When much of the natural crown has been destroyed and the tooth root-filled the crown is made on a core of metal retained by a dowel or post in the root canal.

   These last two types of crown can be used to restore fractured or discoloured teeth or to change the shape, size or position of malformed teeth.

Principles of cavity design for gold inlays

Cavities prepared for gold inlays differ from cavities for plastic filling materials in three main features:

● The cavity must allow withdrawal of the wax pattern and insertion of the restoration in only one direction, the axis of the cavity (Fig. 9.1).
● The cavo-surface angle should be bevelled, where necessary.
● The toughness and high proportional limit of type C gold alloys permit thin extra-coronal extensions of the casting to be used to protect weak tooth substance or to assist in retention.

ACCESS

The main difference in gaining access to caries for an inlay preparation, compared with an amalgam preparation, is that no undercuts should be produced. Extensive use of the tapered fissure bur is indicated.

REMOVAL OF CARIES

This is carried out exactly as for direct restorations. The undercuts which occur as a result of the removal of caries may be eliminated either by cutting back the overhanging part of the tooth or, if confined to the dentine, they may be blocked out by lining material. Cutting back is indicated where the undercut is small or moderate in extent and a combination of cutting back and blocking out is indicated where it is extensive (Fig. 6.1).

BIOLOGICAL FORM

Full extension of the preparation along deep or stained fissures and buccally, lingually and gingivally to clear approximal contacts, is necessary. This approximal extension is also needed, as a matter of convenience, to facilitate finishing the margins of the preparation, taking an impression or wax pattern, checking the fit, and finishing the restoration.

MECHANICAL FORM

Withdrawal Since cast gold is not plastic at mouth temperature, retention cannot be obtained by means of undercuts; in fact undercuts would prevent the removal of the wax pattern and the insertion of the finished casting. It follows that there must be one

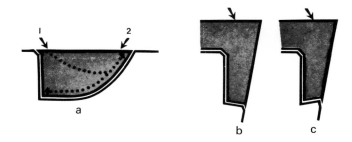

Fig. 9.2 Stability in inlay cavities.
(*a*) The inlay is unstable with respect to force 1 and can be displaced; it cannot be displaced by force 2 because of the vertical wall and the square internal angle.
(*b*) The inlay can be displaced laterally, in the absence of a dovetail, because of the unfavourably sloping gingival floor.
(*c*) The inlay is stable because of the favourably sloping gingival floor.

direction, but only one direction, in which the wax pattern can be removed and the cast gold restoration inserted (Fig. 9.1). This is called the line of withdrawal or *axis* of the cavity. The casting should be vulnerable to displacement only along its axis, and therefore the line of withdrawal should be opposed to the direction of the main functional load. This load then tends to force the casting into the cavity and not to displace it. In complex cavities in particular it is essential to ensure that all parts of the cavity, such as the dovetail and the box, allow withdrawal along the same axis.

Stability   This is provided by flat floors perpendicular to the axis to the cavity, by sharp internal line angles and by favourably sloping floors (Fig. 9.2).

Retention   Resistance to displacement of an inlay along its axis is called *axial retention* whilst resistance to displacement sideways is called *lateral retention* (Fig. 9.3).
  Axial retention is produced by:

- Friction between the casting and the walls of the preparation.
- Cement locking in the micro-irregularities between the casting and the walls

  Axial retention is increased by (Fig. 9.4):

- Nearness to parallel of the opposing walls of the preparation.
- Increase in the area of near-parallel opposing walls (Lorey & Myers 1968).
- Closeness of apposition of the casting to the cavity walls.
- Increase in the strength of the cementing medium.

Since retention is improved by increasing the length of the opposing walls it follows that, in the completed cavity after lining, sharp internal line angles are preferable to the rounded angles which are indicated for plastic fillings. The walls of inlay cavities

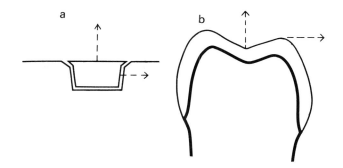

Fig. 9.3 Types of retention required for an inlay (intra-coronal) and a crown (extra-coronal).
(*a*) Axial retention to resist displacement along the axis.
(*b*) Lateral retention to resist sideways displacement and tilt.

converge towards the floor. The line angles around the floor are, therefore, farther away from the pulp horns than in undercut cavities, and the risk of pulpal exposure from sharp internal angles is less. In shallow cavities it is necessary to make the walls nearly parallel and to restrict the bevel to a minimum in order to obtain sufficient retention. With deeper cavities, where a larger area of near-parallel opposing walls is available for retention, these may be allowed to diverge up to 5° to the axis. In fact this is often desirable to allow for operator error in paralleling the walls of complex cavities. The majority of cavities should have walls at an angle of 2.5° to the axis.

Lateral retention can be obtained in inlay cavities by means of dovetails and favourable floor slopes as for direct restorations. In addition, tapered or parallel-sided pin-holes drilled into the dentine parallel to the axis of the cavity, are valuable since the pins, incorporated into the casting, provide both lateral and axial retention. Thin veneers of metal extending extra-coronally may also assist lateral retention.

Marginal finish As is the general rule, sharp angles in the cavity outline should be avoided. The cavo-surface angle should be bevelled, in contrast to the 90° angle preferred in amalgam cavities. A continuous bevel is prepared around the margins of the cavity, gingivally, buccally, lingually and occlusally. Occlusally the bevel angle should be approximately 135° but on the gingival and lingual margins and on those buccal margins which are not normally visible the angle should be greater so as to give a longer flange on the inlay corresponding to the bevel. Where the tooth is strongly convex on its approximal surface great care is needed to ensure that the whole of the bevel will withdraw. The bevel must cut back the tooth contour until no part of it is below the survey line. In situations where aesthetics are important it may be

139   *Inlays and crowns*

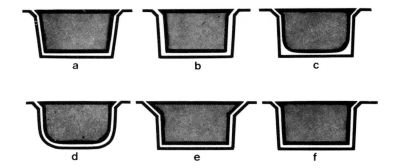

Fig. 9.4 Axial retention of inlays. (*a–e*) These show inadequate retention; only *f* has good retention. In *a* the walls diverge too much; in *b* the inlay does not fit the cavity closely; in *c* the inlay does not fit the internal angles; in *d* the cavity is too rounded; and in *e* the bevel is too extensive. Thus in *c*, *d* and *e* the effective length of the near-parallel opposing walls is reduced.

necessary to modify the bevels of the buccal margins of the cavities in order to show less metal. In very shallow cavities bevels should be minimal in order to increase retention by providing a greater length of cavity wall.

The purpose of the bevel is two-fold. It gives added strength to the enamel margin, which is particularly valuable in a two-stage operation where the removal of a temporary dressing may damage a weak enamel margin and destroy the fit of the inlay. It also provides a tapered flange on the inlay which can be swaged or adapted prior to cementing to improve the marginal fit and correct any minor inaccuracy of the casting (Fig. 9.5) (Christensen 1966). The bevel on an inlay is permissible because of the high strength of gold casting alloys which prevents fracture.

SELECTION OF THE ALLOY

Four types of gold casting alloy are generally available. The softer alloys allow some adaptation or swaging of the margins but may distort if used in load-bearing sites. Type A (soft) is useful for Class V box preparations since there is no occlusal load. Type B (medium) is indicated in intra-coronal cavities. Type C (hard) is used for all veneer preparations including Class V pinlays, inlays bearing rests or clasps of partial dentures, and cusp-covered restorations. Type D (very hard) is not often used for the restoration of individual teeth but sometimes for posts.

Preparations for cast gold inlays

CLASS II

If the carious cavity has already broken through to the occlusal surface access should be obtained at this point. Where an adjacent

Fig. 9.5 Value of a bevel on an inlay cavity.
In *a* there is no possibility of improving the marginal adaptation.
In *b* the flange on the periphery of the inlay can be swaged against the bevel on the cavity margin to improve marginal adaptation.

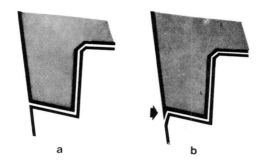

a   b

approximal cavity is being prepared entry should be made directly into the contact area, cutting both approximal surfaces at once. If, however, the adjacent tooth is sound or satisfactorily restored and the caries has not reached the occlusal surface, entry should be made near one or other end of the occlusal fissure using a tapered fissure tungsten carbide or diamond bur. The bur is held at an angle so that its side is used to cut obliquely into the fissure, and gradually brought into a vertical position, as it reaches a depth of about 2.5 mm (Fig. 9.6a). The bur is carried along all the deep and stained fissures at this depth and used to form a T-shape at one end over the site of the approximal caries and a dovetail at the other end (Fig. 9.6b, c). The bur should be held constant in the axis which has been selected for withdrawal. The T-shape should be cut immediately inside the approximal enamel wall extending as far buccally and lingually as the beginning of the embrasures, but over-extension at these points should be avoided. At the other end the dovetail should be prepared well inside the marginal ridge so that this is not weakened. Again, keeping the bur in the same axis, the T-shaped end of the cavity is deepened to a depth just level with the bottom of the contact area (Fig. 9.6d). If the stationary bur is first placed just outside the tooth it can be used to gauge the depth to which the box should be cut at this point.

A hatchet chisel may be used to lever out the weakened wall of enamel (Fig. 9.6e). If the enamel does not fracture easily it should be further weakened using a tapered fissure bur in the T-shaped slot. A hatchet or contra-angle chisel is used to plane the buccal and lingual walls to form an approximal box withdrawable in the same axis as the dovetail (Fig. 9.6f, g).

Caries is removed using a round bur, checking with an excavator to ensure that no soft dentine remains. A base may be inserted at this stage or, if preferred, at the end of the preparation. After the material has set, a tapered fissure bur is used to finish the walls, floors and outline of the occlusal part of the cavity. At the

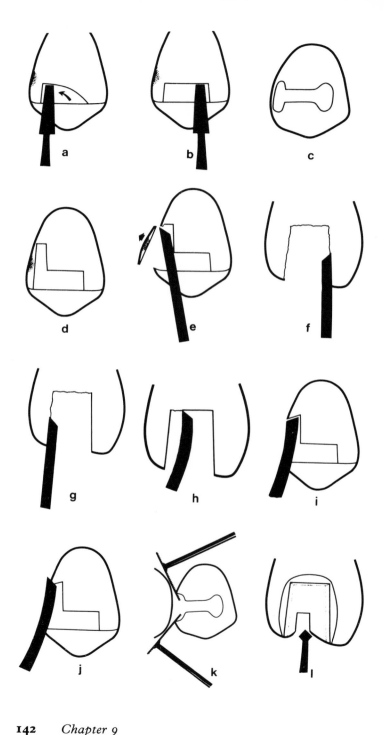

Fig. 9.6 Preparation of a Class II inlay cavity. Details of the stages of preparation are given in the text.

same time the axial wall is smoothed and the approximal box given a precise withdrawable shape. Finally, the bur is used to bevel the axio-pulpal line angle, if this is considered necessary.

A margin trimmer (77/78 in a mesial box and 79/80 in a distal box) is used first to flatten the gingival floor and then to produce a reverse bevel (Figs 9.6i and 4.14). This second stage may be omitted where it is not considered necessary. Next, a second trimmer (79/80 in a mesial box and 77/80 in a distal box) is used to bevel the gingival margin (Fig. 9.6j). It is used with a scraping motion, first one end and then the other, in the direction towards which the concavity of the blade faces. The gingival bevels are carried up on to the buccal and lingual margins.

The buccal and lingual walls of the box are bevelled and finished. Where adequate space is available a tapered fissure tungsten carbide bur is most suitable, but where space is restricted a fine sandpaper disc should be used (Fig. 9.6k). Alternatively, the gingival, buccal and lingual margins may be finished and bevelled with Baker-Curson burs. It is most important to ensure that the whole of the bevel on the buccal and lingual margins is withdrawable since the convexity of the tooth at this point may render this difficult. Finally, the cavo-surface angle of the occlusal part is bevelled, if desired, using a diamond-shaped stone (Fig. 9.6l).

This technique of preparing a Class II cavity makes use of the shape of the bur to produce the basic shape so the bur should always be held in the axis of the cavity. With practice this is not difficult and the stationary bur can be used to check withdrawal.

Where difficulty arises in preparing a dovetail because of the risk of producing excessive weakness, a pin can be used in place of the dovetail to provide lateral retention.

Summary

The essential features of a Class II inlay cavity are as follows:

● All parts of the dovetail and the box are withdrawable along a single axis which will permit the completed inlay to enter the cavity past the adjacent tooth. The walls of the cavity form an angle of approximately 2.5° to this axis. The internal angles between the walls and the floor are sharp.
● The margins of the approximal box buccally, gingivally and lingually are finished in the form of a continuous bevel. All parts of this bevel are withdrawable in the axis of the cavity. The bevel angle is at least 135° but frequently a longer bevel is required. The occlusal part is bevelled, if considered necessary.

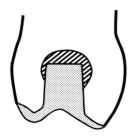

Fig. 9.7 Bucco-lingual cross-section of MOD inlay in upper premolar. The buccal aspect (*right*) shows minimal gold; the lingual cusp (*left*), a supporting cusp, is covered by a thicker layer of metal which has a chamfered margin. The striped area represents a cement base inserted after the removal of caries.

● In other respects the cavity resembles that for a Class II amalgam.

MOD WITH CUSP COVERAGE

This type of preparation is useful where the buccal or lingual cusps have been weakened, usually by caries. Failure to protect weakened cusps may lead to fracture of the whole cusp and the creation of a problem which is less easily solved. The preparation is equally valuable in premolar and molar teeth. The inlay may cover any number of cusps but, generally, if there is a need to protect one, it is wise to consider protecting all from the risk of subsequent fracture.

Before starting the preparation the occlusion must be examined, first in centric occlusion, then in working and non-working side movements and finally in protrusive slide. This will indicate whether the tooth is in balanced occlusion and the areas where cusp reduction is required. The supporting cusps should be covered by 1.5 mm of metal and the remaining cusps by 1 mm in all positions of the occlusion.

Access is obtained and caries removed as described for a Class II inlay. The occlusal preparation is begun in the same manner but boxes are prepared mesially and distally. Great care should be taken to ensure that both boxes allow withdrawal along the same axis. Cusp reduction is begun by making depth orientation grooves on the central slopes of the buccal and lingual cusps using a diamond fissure bur. Two or three grooves are placed on each cusp to a depth of 1.5 mm on the supporting cusps and 1 mm on the remaining cusps. Using these as guides the cusp slopes are reduced by the amount indicated and parallel to the original slope. All positions of the occlusion are checked to ensure that there is adequate clearance. On the buccal cusp this can be done visually, but the lingual cusps may be difficult to see and here it is necessary to use a piece of sheet wax to record occlusion. When held up to the light this will indicate any areas of inadequate clearance. A bevel is placed on the outside of the buccal and lingual cusps. This is small on the buccal cusp of upper teeth to avoid any unnecessary appearance of gold and since these are not usually supporting cusps. On the supporting cusps the bevel should be more pronounced and should end in a definite finishing line (Fig. 9.7). This usually involves the buccal cusps of the lower teeth and the palatal cusps of the upper, where appearance is not so important. These bevels are extended to become continuous with those on the mesial and distal surfaces.

Fig. 9.8 Cavity preparation for a Class V inlay.
(a) Cross-section showing the carious lesion before treatment; (b) removal of caries with a large round bur; (c) preparation of the box form using a tapered or parallel-sided plain-cut bur; (d) bevelling the enamel cavo-surface angle lightly; (e) longitudinal section showing the completed cavity.

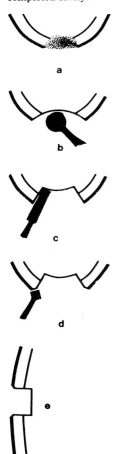

Summary

The essential features of an MOD inlay cavity with cusp coverage are as follows:

● All parts of each box and the occlusal section are withdrawable in the same axis.
● The supporting cusps are 1.5 mm, and the non-supporting cusps 1 mm, clear of the opposing teeth in all occlusal movements.
● The marginal finish and internal form is as described for a Class II cavity.

CLASS V

There are two basic forms of cavity preparation for a Class V inlay, one a box-shaped preparation and the second making use of pins to provide retention and stability. A combination of these techniques is possible.

The box-shaped preparation is more suitable where caries is present in the dentine and comparatively little removal of sound dentine is required. The pin-retained inlay is indicated where the cavity is wide and does not penetrate deeply into the dentine as in cases of abrasion and erosion.

Box preparation

Access is not a problem because the thin layer of enamel overlying the cavity is quickly broken down. The caries is removed by means of a large round bur (Fig. 9.8). A plain-cut tungsten carbide fissure bur is used to develop a retentive box by maintaining the bur at a depth of 1.5–2 mm and moving it in such a way that its long axis remains perpendicular to the surface of the tooth; the occlusal and gingival walls should be very slightly divergent towards the surface. If the tooth surface is flat the mesial and distal may also be parallel but, if the tooth is curved, the mesial and distal walls will diverge and the floor of the cavity will be convex. The main retention is then obtained between the gingival and occlusal walls. A stationary bur should be used to check the withdrawal form of the cavity.

Finally, the whole of the cavo-surface angle of the cavity is bevelled, using a diamond-shaped stone, but the bevel is kept small in order to avoid reducing the retention. Sub-gingivally,

145 *Inlays and crowns*

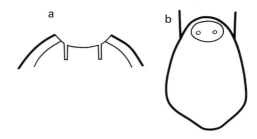

Fig. 9.9 Completed preparation for a Class V pin-retained inlay. (*a*) Cross-section; (*b*) labial view.

retraction fibre will give good access during the use of hand instruments or the making of a wax pattern. If the cavity extends far sub-gingivally some gingival tissue will have to be removed. Electrosurgery provides a convenient means of doing this (Chapter 12).

Summary The essential features of a Class V inlay box preparation cavity are as follows:

● All parts of the cavity are withdrawable along a single axis. The incisal or occlusal wall and the gingival wall are parallel or nearly so. Where the cavity is on a curved surface the mesial and distal walls diverge and run approximately radially. Where the cavity is on a flat surface the mesial and distal walls may be nearly parallel.
● There is a slight bevel on the cavo-surface angle around the whole periphery.

Pin-retained preparation

Caries, if present, is removed with a round bur leaving a shallow concave depression. This depression is extended by means of a round diamond instrument until all carious enamel has been removed and an adequate depth achieved at the sites of the proposed pins and around the margins. The pins should be placed mesially and distally so that the holes are midway between the pulp and the enamel–dentine junction and midway between the occlusal and gingival margins. The pin-holes are started with a No. $\frac{1}{2}$ round bur and their positions assessed. The holes are then drilled to a depth of about 2.5 mm in an axis parallel to one another using an 0.6 mm twist drill. They must be drilled with precision so that they are absolutely parallel (Fig. 9.9).

Principles of design for crown preparations

BIOLOGICAL FORM

This is mainly concerned with the position of the margins in relation to the gingival crest. If caries or an existing restoration has already extended sub-gingivally the crown must, where possible, be carried beyond this on to sound tooth tissue. In all other cases the margin should be at the same level as the gingival crest, where appearance is important, or slightly supra-gingival where it is not. The fit and finish should be as good as possible to minimise the permanent gingival damage and permit plaque removal by the patient. The key to good gingival health around crowns is to establish a high standard of oral hygiene, including interdental hygiene, before treatment is begun, to achieve a well-contoured and well-fitting restoration and to place the margins supra-gingivally where possible. This is discussed at greater length in Chapter 12.

MECHANICAL FORM

Withdrawal As with inlays, preparations for crowns must be free from undercuts and allow withdrawal of the crown along the axis of the preparation.

Stability This is derived from flat surfaces opposing the direction of load and these may be on the occlusal surfaces, incisal edges or shoulders of the preparation. Well-defined shoulders are particularly important in porcelain jacket crowns, which may crack if the load is not evenly spread.

Retention *Axial* retention and *lateral* retention are obtained in the same way as for inlays and so the preparation for a crown should have sufficient area of near-parallel opposing walls to give adequate retention (Fig. 9.3). Where these are not available in natural tooth substance they may be provided in the form of a core or the root canal may be used.

Thickness During the preparation, sufficient tooth substance must be removed to provide enough thickness in the finished crown. This is needed to give strength, especially in the weaker materials such as porcelain.

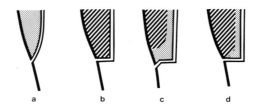

Fig. 9.10 Marginal finish of crown preparations: (*a*) chamfered margin for full veneer cast gold crown; (*b*) shoulder for porcelain crown; (*c*) bevelled wide shoulder for porcelain bonded to metal crown with metal collar; (*d*) wide shoulder for porcelain bonded to metal crown.

Marginal finish

The shape of the margins of the preparation dictates the shape of the finished restoration and therefore must be related to the properties of the materials which are to be used. Cast gold has a high proportional limit and so can be used in comparatively thin layers, as with chamfered margins (Fig. 9.10a). This is the recommended finish for full veneer gold crowns. It is superior to a knife-edge since it gives a clear indication to the technician as to where the wax pattern should be finished and avoids having to work with a thin edge of wax from which small pieces may fracture. It gives adequate thickness of metal at the margin of the finished crown, without the need to overcontour it, yet with some degree of bevel which enables a better fit to be obtained.

Porcelain, on the other hand, is weak in thin layers and so the margin for a porcelain crown must be in the shape of a square shoulder with no bevel so that an adequate bulk of material is present (Fig. 9.10b).

In porcelain bonded to metal crowns several types of finish are used. Where the porcelain is to be kept far away from the gingival margin and metal only extended to this level, a chamfer finishing line is used. Where the porcelain is to be extended to, or close to, the margin of the crown, sufficient space must be obtained to accommodate it. A shoulder at least 1.5 mm and preferably 2 mm wide is needed to give an adequate thickness for the cement, metal and overlying porcelain. Greater strength and a better fit is provided where the casting is present in bulk at the gingival margin so that a collar of metal shows around the whole periphery of the crown (Fig. 9.10c). This requires the preparation of a bevelled shoulder. It is indicated on lingual surfaces, and on buccal surfaces which are not aesthetically important such as upper and lower molars and most lower premolars, canines and incisors. It is not usually acceptable in upper incisors, canines and premolars where the margin is often visible during lip movements. Here it is necessary to finish the preparation as a shoulder without a bevel; a thin layer of metal will extend almost to the surface and be covered by porcelain so that it is completely masked (Fig. 9.10d). At least 1.5 mm of tissue must be removed to give adequate thickness for the cement, metal and overlying porcelain.

Preparations for crowns

Preparatory stages

Often the tooth to be prepared has already been extensively affected by caries and it may have already been restored. The status of the pulp must be investigated and the operator must be assured that either the pulp is healthy or the tooth is satisfactorily root filled. The loss of tooth substance may have affected the available retention and this must be corrected by building a core which can be used to provide retention and stability for the crown. Unless he knows that the pulp condition is satisfactory, that all necessary caries has been removed and that the existing restoration will still have adequate retention after the preparation of the crown, the careful operator will wish to remove existing restorations, explore beneath them and replace them by a stable core. In posterior teeth the core is formed of amalgam or composite material and retained by pins where necessary (Chapter 7). In anterior teeth it is usual to build a core, retained by a post in the root canal, as described later in this chapter. However, it is possible to use a pin-retained composite core in anterior teeth and to use some form of post retention in posterior teeth.

Study casts are essential prior to the construction of crowns. They have the following functions:

- As pre-operative records for later comparison.
- For modelling any proposed changes.
- To permit a better examination of the occlusion.
- To form a matrix for making temporary crowns.
- For construction of a special tray.

Before commencing, the operator must be assured that the gingival health is good and that the patient will maintain this by effective oral hygiene. He must inspect the occlusion in all functional movements and determine how much of the crown of the tooth is visible during talking and smiling. This information will help him to plan precisely the type of crown he will use and the amount of tooth reduction required.

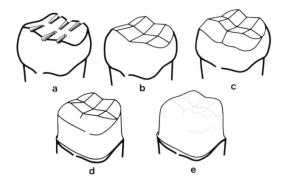

Fig. 9.11 Stages in the preparation of a molar tooth for a full veneer gold cast crown: (*a*) depth orientation grooves occlusally; (*b*) reduction of occlusal surface; (*c*) reduction of occlusal part of buccal and lingual sides; (*d*) mesial, distal, buccal and lingual sides prepared, with chamfer finish gingivally; (*e*) completed preparation smoothed and rounded.

Full veneer gold crown

The first stage is the reduction of the occlusal surface, since after this is completed the operator is able to determine the available retention. The prepared occlusal surface must be at least 1.5 mm clear of the opposing teeth on the supporting cusps (that is the buccal of the lower teeth and the palatal of the upper in a normal occlusion), and 1 mm clear on the non-supporting cusps, in any functional position. A diamond fissure bur 1.5 mm in diameter should be used to make several depth orientation grooves of the required depth on the occlusal fissures and ridges, to give a clear indication of how much tooth substance needs to be removed (Fig. 9.11a). This will save repeated checks of the occlusion. The remaining occlusal surface is reduced using a round-ended tapered diamond bur and following the contour of the occlusal slopes on the original tooth surface (Fig. 9.11b). This ensures that an even, adequate thickness is removed without excessive loss of tooth substance and retention (Fig. 9.12). The preparation should be stopped just short of the contact areas to avoid damage to the adjacent teeth; this part will be removed later.

The second stage is to reduce the outward-facing slopes of the cusps with the same diamond bur (Fig. 9.11c). This reduction will be more extensive on the supporting cusps than on the others. This important stage is necessary to give sufficient thickness for the crown; if it is not done it may be impossible for the technician to construct the crown with a balanced occlusion and certainly he will have to make it abnormally wide occlusally. The occlusal clearance in functional movements can usually be seen on the buccal cusps but, as described earlier, the lingual cusps may need to be checked with a small sheet of wax to ensure that there is adequate clearance.

Next, the mesial and distal contacts are reduced using a

Fig. 9.12 Unsatisfactory preparations for full veneer cast gold crowns. In (*a*) the walls converge too strongly giving poor retention and resistance to tilt; in (*b*) the cusps have been flattened excessively reducing the height of the preparation and its axial retention; in (*c*) the natural crown is very short and so the preparation should have near-parallel sides, to get maximum retention, with some intra-coronal retention added; in (*d*) the occlusal surface and occlusal parts of the buccal and lingual surfaces have not been sufficiently reduced and so the crown cannot be made thick enough; (*e*) shows the correct preparation.

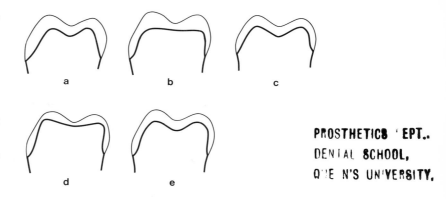

round-ended tapered diamond bur and cutting into the tooth surface sufficiently far to ensure that no damage is done to the adjacent tooth or restoration. The reduction should extend from buccal to lingual and sufficiently far gingivally to clear the contact with the adjacent tooth. The same bur is used to extend the approximal preparation on to and along the buccal and lingual surfaces, providing sufficient convergence to give adequate retention and yet ensure withdrawal. The junctions between the axial walls should be rounded, following the contour of the tooth and completing a continuous chamfer around the whole of the gingival margin of the preparation (Fig. 9.11d). Finally, the preparation should be smoothed with a fine sandpaper disc (Fig. 9.11e).

Summary

The essential features of the preparation for a full veneer gold crown are as follows:

● There should be a continuous chamfer around the whole of the margin. This should extend slightly beyond the limits of any core but otherwise it should be kept at, or slightly above, the level of the gingival crest.
● The mesial and distal walls and the gingival parts of the buccal and lingual walls should converge sufficiently to give withdrawal form yet provide adequate retention.
● The supporting cusps should be 1.5 mm clear of the opposing cusps in all functional movements and the non-supporting cusps should be 1 mm clear.
● The outer slopes of the cusps should be reduced sufficiently to

provide adequate thickness of crown without the need to develop excessive contour in the finished crown.

Full veneer porcelain bonded to metal crown—molar and premolar teeth

The principles involved in this preparation are the same as those for the full veneer gold crown and similar burs and cutting techniques are used. The differences lie in the greater thickness required for the combination of porcelain and metal, and in the distribution of these two materials at the marginal areas of the crown. The whole of the prepared surface of the tooth will be covered by metal. In the case of molars and premolars the occlusal surface, most of the buccal surface as far round as the beginning of the contact areas and the occlusal part of the lingual surface will have porcelain overlying the metal. The gingival half of the lingual surface and the contact areas will be finished in metal without any superimposed porcelain. A metal-to-tooth margin gives a better fit than a porcelain-to-tooth margin and is desirable, even on the buccal surface, in the form of a collar of metal (Fig 9.10c). Unfortunately, this is generally unacceptable in areas which are seen and here a compromise is reached in the form of a porcelain-to-tooth margin with the porcelain supported underneath by metal (Fig 9.10d).

The preparation is commenced as for a full veneer gold crown by reducing the occlusal surface, but an extra 0.5 mm must be removed to allow for the combined thickness of the porcelain and metal. The supporting cusps must therefore be reduced by at least 2 mm and the non-supporting cusps by 1.5 mm. The buccal reduction of the finished preparation must allow 1.5–2 mm thickness for metal and porcelain.

After the occlusal reduction has been completed the outer slopes of the cusps are reduced. The mesial, lingual and distal surfaces are prepared in the same manner as for a full veneer gold crown but making sure that an adequate depth of tooth substance is removed.

The buccal reduction must extend into the embrasures and particularly the mesial embrasure. Where a metal-to-tooth margin is planned buccally a bevelled shoulder of the appropriate depth is prepared. Baker-Curson burs are ideal for finishing this. Where a porcelain-to-tooth margin is necessary a shoulder without a bevel is produced. It is most important to remove sufficient tooth otherwise the overlying porcelain may be too thin and may give a poor appearance due to the opaque layer showing through the

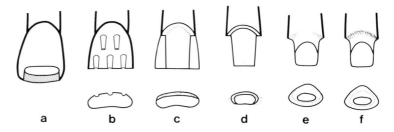

Fig. 9.13 Stages in the preparation of an upper central incisor for a porcelain bonded to gold crown; (*a*) removal of incisal edge; (*b*) depth orientation grooves; (*c*) labial surface and gingival shoulder; (*d*) proximal surfaces; (*e*) lingual fossa; and (*f*) lingual wall and chamfer.

overlying dentine layer. If the tooth will not permit this degree of reduction then it must be considered unsuitable for this type of crown.

Summary

The important features of the preparation for a full veneer porcelain bonded to metal crown are as follows:

● Sufficient tooth substance must be removed to permit a minimum thickness of crown of 1.5 mm. On the supporting cusps, and if possible buccally, the crown should be 2 mm thick.
● A chamfered finishing line of slightly greater depth than for a gold crown is required mesially, distally and lingually. A square shoulder is prepared on the buccal surface, extending into the mesial and distal embrasures, where a porcelain-to-tooth margin has been selected; for a metal-to-tooth margin a bevelled shoulder is required.
● The other features are similar to the preparation for a full veneer gold crown.

Full veneer porcelain bonded to metal crown—incisor and canine teeth.

The technique is described for upper teeth; for lower teeth the principles are similar but the occlusion is reversed and it may be more difficult to achieve the recommended clearances. The first stage in the preparation is to reduce the incisal edge by 2.5–3 mm or, more correctly, to a line which is this distance from the incisal edge of the finished crown (Fig. 9.13a). The side of a diamond fissure bur is entered into the labial face at this level and carried mesially and distally to produce a groove. This groove is gradually deepened and extended through to the lingual surface until the incisal portion is held in position only by a thin piece of tooth mesially and distally. At this stage it can readily be broken off, leaving the adjacent teeth undamaged.

Preparation of the labial surface commences by cutting several depth orientation grooves in the incisal part and again on the gingival part (Fig. 9.13b). The surface is generally convex and this shape should be maintained in the finished preparation. The grooves should be at least 1.5 mm deep and this can be checked since the diameter of the bur is known. The grooves are joined together, first the incisal grooves and then the gingival grooves, so that the required depth of tooth substance is removed. If the tooth surface is simply worn down by grinding, all trace of depth will soon be lost and the finished preparation may easily be too shallow or too deep. There should now be a square shoulder just above the level of the gingivae (Fig. 9.13c).

The labial reduction is extended mesially and distally so as to continue the shoulder through the contacts, just supra-gingivally, and with a slight convergence of these walls towards the incisal edge, avoiding damage to the adjacent teeth. The preparation is extended as far lingually as direct vision will allow (Fig. 9.13d).

Continuing to use a flat-ended diamond fissure bur, the labial surface is smoothed and sharp angles between labial and approximal surfaces are rounded. The labial shoulder is extended until it is level with the gingival crest, is of adequate width and has a 90° angle with the axial walls. Where appearance is most important this shoulder is taken a fraction of a millimetre sub-gingivally; where it is not, the shoulder is left just supra-gingivally.

Reduction of the lingual surface is commenced using a small diamond wheel at high speed on the lingual fossa and reducing this until it is 1–1.5 mm clear of the opposing teeth in centric occlusion, right and left lateral movements and protrusive slide (Fig. 9.13e). The preparation of the lingual gingival margin is best carried out by direct vision, with the chair almost horizontal and the headrest tilted backwards. Using a round-ended tapered diamond fissure bur the shoulder on the labial half of the tooth is continued just supra-gingivally along the whole of the lingual margin in the form of a deep chamfer (Fig. 9.13f). The short lingual wall is aligned so that it converges slightly in relation to the labial surface to achieve a withdrawable shape. The chamfer should be continuous with the mesial and distal shoulders to form a single smooth curve.

Finally, the preparation should be generally smoothed, sharp angles removed and the gingival shoulder accentuated where necessary to form a 90° angle. Where a metal collar is being used at the labial gingival margin a bevel is superimposed on the shoulder. Baker-Curson burs of appropriate shapes are ideal for these finishing procedures. Where it is not possible to obtain sufficient clearance on the lingual surface for both metal and porcelain the porcelain is omitted from this area and finished nearer the incisal edge.

Summary

The following are the main features of a full veneer porcelain bonded to metal crown on an anterior tooth:

● There must be a clearance of 1.5 mm between the lingual surface of an upper anterior preparation and the opposing lower teeth, or 0.5 mm for metal only, and a clearance of 2.5–3 mm incisally.
● There must be room for a thickness of at least 1.5 mm labially and preferably more. One of the most common errors in anterior crown preparation is a failure to remove sufficient tooth substance from the labial surface near the incisal edge. This mistake leads to an inadequate thickness of porcelain covering the opaque layer and results in a poor appearance.
● Otherwise the same principles apply as for a similar crown on a posterior tooth.

Porcelain jacket crown

Incisal edge reduction is carried out as described above so that the preparation is 2–3 mm short of the position of the incisal edge of the finished crown. Depth orientation grooves are placed on the labial surface, 2 or 3 grooves on the incisal part and 2 or 3 grooves in the gingival part to a depth of 1 mm. These are used as a guide to the reduction of the labial surface which is carried out with a flat-ended diamond fissure bur, forming a square shoulder just supra-gingivally and retaining the natural curvature of the labial surface.

The approximal reduction is made with the same bur carrying the shoulder through the mesial and distal contacts, being careful to avoid any damage to the adjacent teeth, and producing a slight convergence towards the incisal edge. The mesial and distal shoulders are continued lingually as far as possible by direct vision, looking between the teeth.

The lingual surface is best prepared by direct vision with the chair nearly horizontal and head tilted backwards. Reduction of the lingual fossa is carried out using a small diamond wheel at high speed until there is a clearance of at least 1 mm from the opposing teeth in all functional movements. The gingival shoulder is carried round the lingual margin just supra-gingivally, maintaining the

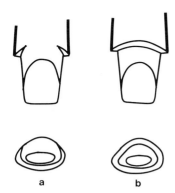

Fig 9.14 Lingual view of the final stages of preparation for a porcelain jacket crown; (*a*) preparation of the area of the lingual fossa; (*b*) preparation of the lingual shoulder.

1 mm width of the shoulder and the 90° angle with the axial walls. The short lingual wall is aligned so as to converge slightly with the labial surface (Fig. 9.14).

All sharp projecting angles on the preparation are gently rounded and the gingival shoulder is emphasised with a cylindrical Baker-Curson bur, maintaining the shoulder supra-gingivally on the lingual half of the tooth, but at gingival level or very slightly sub-gingivally on the labial half where appearance requires this.

Summary

The important features of a preparation of an anterior tooth for a porcelain jacket crown are:

● There is a 1 mm shoulder all around the preparation, supra-gingivally on the lingual half of the tooth, and at or slightly sub-gingivally on the labial half where appearance demands.
● There is convergence of mesial and distal, and labial and lingual pairs of axial walls, sufficient to permit insertion of the crown, yet maintaining adequate retention.
● An adequate depth of tooth substance is removed to permit at least 1 mm thickness of porcelain in all areas.
● The junctions of the different surfaces are gently rounded since square outlines in the preparation lead to sharp angles within the crown, where crack propagation is likely to commence.

Post-retained crowns

Extensive damage of the natural crown of a tooth leads to problems of retention. In posterior teeth, and sometimes in anterior teeth, this can be solved by the use of dentine pins for retention of a core of amalgam or composite material (Fig. 9.15a). However, in many cases caries has involved the pulp, and the tooth has been root filled, so it is convenient to use the root canal for retention of the artificial crown, particularly in teeth with single straight canals. This need should be foreseen before the root filling is carried out so that a technique can be used which will allow subsequent use of the canal for retention. This generally means that the apical third of the canal is filled by an endodontic point and sealer, and the remaining two-thirds by material which can subsequently be removed without disturbing the apical seal.

The method of using the canal for retention involves the construction of a piece of metal which extends sufficiently far into the canal to give stability and retention, and which at the coronal

Fig. 9.15 Methods of building up a core on an upper incisor tooth prior to crowning: (*a*) composite core retained by dentine pins, on vital tooth; (*b*) cast post and core; (*c*) Wiptam wrought post and cast core; (*d*) prefabricated post and core—Charlton type; (*e*) prefabricated threaded post and core—Kurer type. In *b*, *c*, *d* and *e*, a root filling has been placed prior to crowning.

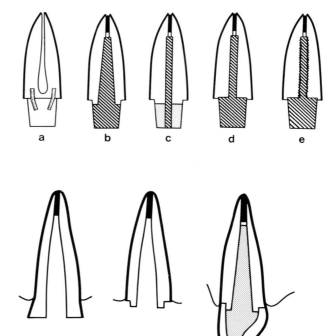

a   b   c   d   e

Fig. 9.16 Preparation of tooth for a cast post and core porcelain jacket crown in root-filled tooth. (*a*) and (*b*) are mesio-distal views; (*c*) is a bucco-lingual view. (*a*) preparation of canal; (*b*) preparation of root face; (*c*) completed porcelain jacket crown with cast post and core.

a   b   c

end is shaped into a core resembling the preparation for a veneer crown (Fig. 9.16). The post should be at least as long as the crown of the tooth, to give adequate retention and resistance, and longer if possible. This post and core is cemented into the canal and the crown is cemented on to the core. The crown and core should not be made in one piece, otherwise renewal of the crown at a future date becomes unnecessarily difficult and hazardous, but an exception may be made in small-crowned teeth where space may not permit this. During the preparation great care should be taken to avoid penetrating the wall of the canal.

There are two types of post and core; the first is constructed specifically for the preparation and the second is prefabricated.

POST AND CORE—LABORATORY MADE

This technique is suitable for almost all situations but, since it is constructed specifically for the prepared tooth, it is especially suitable for atypical cases. For example, if caries or a fracture has taken the root face sub-gingivally a complete or partial diaphragm may be incorporated.

In preparing the root face it is wise to preserve any useful dentine which remains supra-gingivally. The preparation begins by entering the side of a diamond fissure bur into the labial surface of the crown at least 2 mm above the level of the interdental papillae. The cut is carried through to the lingual surface and extended mesially and distally until the remaining tooth is so weak that it can be split off without damage to the adjacent teeth. The labial, lingual and approximal surfaces are now prepared, as for a porcelain jacket crown, or porcelain bonded to metal crown, whichever is being used. Using a face-cutting diamond stone at low speed, or a diamond fissure bur at high speed, the incisal edge is flattened until it is judged that the dentine core, left after preparation of the canal, will be adequately strong.

Cast post and core (Fig. 9.15b)

The canal is prepared to a tapered shape. Access is re-established into the root canal with a round bur and the preparation is completed with a tapered fissure bur used at low speed so that the canal has a gentle taper. A small anti-rotational groove is cut into a strong part of the dentine, unless the canal is already eccentric. An impression is taken in an appropriate elastic material, syringing it into the canal and placing in it a length of wire to give it rigidity before seating the impression tray. In the laboratory the technician will construct a die, use it to form a wax pattern of the post and core and cast this in gold. A non-precious metal may be used provided it will not be exposed in the mouth. This technique is not so satisfactory in slender teeth such as lower incisors since a narrow cast post will be weak, the impression technique more difficult and widening the canal may result in weakening of the tooth.

Where several posts and cores are being made by the indirect method it is better to cement these and take a new impression, since the root canals may not be in alignment and this may lead to inaccuracies in the impression and affect the fit of the finished crowns. In some cases it may be more appropriate to construct the pattern for the post and core in the mouth, using wax or a suitable resin, and to have this cast in the laboratory.

Wiptam technique (Fig. 9.15c)

This makes use of a prefabricated post of Wiptam wire, a cobalt chrome alloy, but the core is constructed for the individual tooth. The canal is widened up to a diameter of 1 mm using endodontic reamers to a length just short of the apical part of the root filling. It is further enlarged by hand using a series of twist drills in diameter 1.05 mm, 1.15 mm, 1.25 mm, 1.35 mm and 1.55 mm. The canal should be enlarged only to the size necessary to give the post adequate support. The canal usually widens at its coronal end and this part must be prepared to a withdrawable shape with a tapered fissure bur and a small anti-rotational groove cut into the strongest part of the dentine, generally the lingual side.

A piece of Wiptam wire, 0.05 mm less than the diameter of the largest twist drill used, is prepared by slightly rounding one end which is then seated in the canal. The other end is marked level with the incisal edge of the adjacent teeth, removed from the tooth and sectioned at the mark. It is replaced in the canal and an impression taken in an elastic material, injecting the material around the sides of the post as far as it will go. In the laboratory the technician constructs the die, places the Wiptam wire, shortens it until it is level with the proposed incisal edge of the finished core and notches the part which will project from the canal. The core and the wide part of the canal are built up in wax, invested, and metal is cast on to the post. Sometimes it may be considered appropriate to build up the core in the mouth using wax or an appropriate burn-out resin prior to having this cast in the laboratory.

POST AND CORE—PREFABRICATED TYPE

These techniques involve the preparation of a parallel-sided canal to a standard diameter with standardised preparation of the root face.

The *Charlton* system makes use of a stainless steel post and core available in a number of sizes (Fig. 9.15d). The canal is prepared to the required length with a fissure bur, preceded by a round bur, using low speed. The root face is slotted with a diamond wheel to allow the core to seat and to prevent rotation. The core must be shaped outside the mouth to provide the correct contour for subsequent crowning. At this stage it is cemented and the operator can proceed to construct the crown. The system encourages the use of large posts, the removal of all supra-gingival dentine and tends to be rather destructive.

The *Kurer* post is in the form of a parallel-sided screw (Fig. 9.15e). The canal is prepared to the appropriate size with engine reamers, a root-facer is used to countersink a foundation for the core in the root face, and a special hand tool is used to tap a thread on the wall of the canal. The post and core is screwed in and the length of the post adjusted until the core seats firmly in the prepared foundation. It is then removed and, after isolating and drying the tooth, the post is dipped in cement and screwed home. After the cement has set the core, which is of a softer metal, is trimmed to the required shape with rotary instruments. This form of post gives excellent retention and is particularly useful where only a short length of canal is available, but it is not suitable for wide canals.

Tapered screw posts are sometimes used to augment retention but, since no thread is prepared in the wall of the canal, there is a danger of internal stresses being set up when the post is screwed into position and this may lead to fracture of the root.

REMOVAL OF UNSATISFACTORY RESTORATIONS

It is sometimes necessary to remove an existing inlay or crown prior to remaking it. If the crown or inlay has a margin which is proud it is worth while using a strong instrument, such as a Mitchell's trimmer, with a suitable fulcrum and attempting to lever it out. It is always wise to protect the pharynx in case the restoration comes out suddenly. Great care must be taken to avoid fracturing any weak parts of the tooth. Quite often this approach is ineffective and recourse may have to be made to one of the numerous proprietary crown or bridge removers.

If the restoration still does not come out then it must be sectioned along suitable lines with a diamond or steel fissure bur and removed in several pieces. A Class II inlay might be sectioned at the junction between the approximal and occlusal parts after which the approximal part at least can usually be levered out carefully. In other cases it may be best to cut out the metal along one margin and use this as a fulcrum for levering out the remainder of the restoration along its axis.

Porcelain jacket crowns are easily removed by using a diamond bur at high speed to make a cut axially down the labial surface and through the incisal edge. The crown is then split by inserting an instrument resembling a screw driver into the incisal notch and twisting it carefully. A similar technique can be used for removing full veneer gold crowns and porcelain bonded to metal crowns, but there is greater difficulty in cutting the metal.

In all cases the operator must take great care to use only well-controlled force and to avoid the risk of fracturing thin portions of the remaining tooth substance.

Fig. 9.17 Direct and indirect techniques of inlay construction. *Direct method:* (*a*) cavity in tooth; (*b*) wax pattern in tooth (*c*) completed inlay in tooth. *Indirect method:* (*a*) cavity in tooth; (*d*) impression of tooth; (*e*) model or die of tooth; (*f*) wax pattern and later cast inlay, in model; (*c*) completed inlay in tooth.

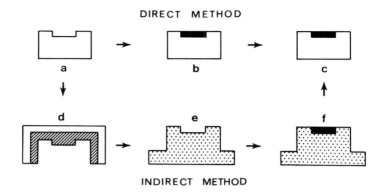

INDIRECT METHOD

It may sometimes be desired to remove a cast post and core or a fractured post. A radiograph will give some indication of the length and retention of the post and of the thickness of the remaining root substance. If there seems a danger of fracturing the root some other approach should be sought. If there seems a good chance of removing the post without damage to the root a post-remover may prove useful. These take various forms; one type has a mechanism for gripping the part of the post projecting from the canal and at the same time drawing the tightly held post from the canal by gradual pressure on the root face using a screw mechanism.

TEMPORARY RESTORATIONS

The construction of an indirect restoration, such as a crown or inlay, involves a period of time, between the preparation of the tooth and the insertion of the completed restoration, during which it is necessary to place a temporary restoration. Temporary crowns and restorations are discussed in Chapter 6.

Construction of an inlay or crown

Before being cast an inlay or metal crown must be formed in wax, or a suitable alternative material, to the precise shape which it is desired that the metal should take. The restoration is then cast using the 'lost wax' process. The wax pattern, as it is called, may be fabricated directly on the tooth in the mouth, or on a model or die in the laboratory. The former is known as the *direct* method and the latter the *indirect* method (Fig. 9.17). The model is obtained from an accurate impression taken in the mouth. The direct method is used with simple, accessible cavities. The indirect technique is indicated for complex cavities and all crowns.

DIRECT TECHNIQUE

Since this technique is becoming less frequently used it will be described only for a box type Class V cavity. Wax is best softened in a wax heater or, failing this, with great care over a flame. In the latter technique, the stick of wax is held some inches above a small flame and is rotated continuously until it becomes thoroughly and homogeneously softened to a state where is can be readily moulded. Overheating to the extent of melting the wax is contra-indicated. The cavity is isolated, dried and painted sparingly with a separating medium. The wax is softened, moulded to a point and forced into the cavity using a plastic-filling instrument and finger pressure and held in position until the wax is set. Excess wax is removed using a wax carver until the required contour is reached and the surface is polished with a dental napkin. The pattern is sprued using a 1.5-mm sprue where possible, or a 1-mm sprue where there is a risk that the margins may be damaged by the larger one. After cooling to mouth temperature the sprue and pattern are removed with great care and checked carefully to ensure that:

● The wax has penetrated completely into the depths of the cavity.
● The margins are intact, particularly the flange corresponding to the bevel on the cavity.
● The sprue is firmly attached to the pattern.

If difficulty is experienced in withdrawing the pattern the cavity should be inspected for undercuts. Another reason for failure of a wax pattern to withdraw is insufficient separating medium. When the pattern is satisfactory, a temporary dressing is placed in the cavity and the patient is discharged. Wax patterns should always be invested as soon as possible.

INDIRECT TECHNIQUE

The first phase in the indirect technique involves the production of a dimensionally accurate impression of the cavity and the adjacent teeth, an impression of the opposing teeth and a record of the occlusion. From these are fabricated models with the aid of which the cast restoration can be constructed. There are many variations of the indirect technique and the method to be described is only one of a number which have given a high degree of success. It involves the production of full arch upper and lower impressions from which models are cast in dental stone with removable precision-fitting dies of the teeth to be restored.

Fig. 9.18 Sectioned impression tray in position on a study cast. Note the space between the tray and the model except where an occlusal stop is present (*arrow*).

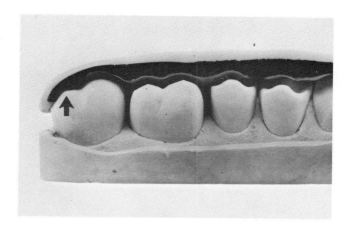

SPECIAL TRAY

A special tray is prepared from a full arch model obtained from a preliminary alginate impression. The teeth and alveolar processes are covered with a spacing material 2–3 mm thick. Spacer is omitted from these areas not involving prepared occlusal surfaces, generally both last molar teeth and the incisal region, in order to build stops into the tray so that it will seat only to the required extent (Fig. 9.18). Acrylic tray material is mixed and moulded by hand into a U-shaped section to cover the buccal, occlusal and lingual surfaces of the teeth. The material is drawn out into handles to facilitate its subsequent removal from the mouth. After the tray material has set, it is removed from the model and the spacing material cleared from it. The periphery is checked to ascertain that it extends a few millimetres beyond the gingival margins of the teeth being restored and it is then trimmed and smoothed with rotary grinding instruments.

A tray for buccal Class V cavities covers that surface of the tooth and gingival tissues, has localising stops on the adjacent teeth and handle. An adequate length of handle, set at the correct angle is particularly necessary on posterior teeth.

IMPRESSION TECHNIQUE

At the chairside, the tray is tried in the mouth, to ensure that it is a satisfactory fit, removed and dried. The whole of the inner surface and the margins are coated with the adhesive designed to be used with the selected impression material and, after this has dried, the tray is ready for use. All haemorrhage should be effectively

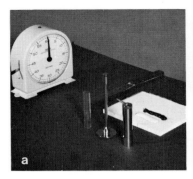
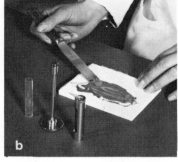
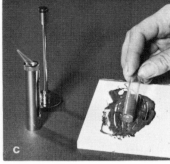
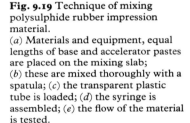
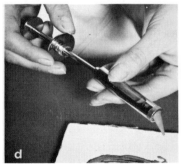

Fig. 9.19 Technique of mixing polysulphide rubber impression material.
(*a*) Materials and equipment, equal lengths of base and accelerator pastes are placed on the mixing slab;
(*b*) these are mixed thoroughly with a spatula; (*c*) the transparent plastic tube is loaded; (*d*) the syringe is assembled; (*e*) the flow of the material is tested.

controlled, if necessary by the use of astringent chemicals or electrosurgery, and the prepared cavity isolated and dried, since the presence of blood or moisture will lead to a deficient impression. Gingival retraction fibre is placed so as to dilate the gingival sulcus adjacent to the cavity margins and is left in position for 3 or 4 minutes after which time the mixing of the impression materials is begun (Fig. 9.19). When mixing is nearly completed the retraction fibre is removed and the cavity redried. The syringe containing the light-bodied impression material is used to inject first into the gingival sulcus (Fig. 9.20) and, by moving the nozzle of the syringe around the approximal box and the occlusal section while slowly injecting, the cavity is filled from inside to outside. Only sufficient material is used to fill the cavity and cover the margins; this is particularly important in the upper arch, where excess light-bodied material will slump out of the cavity and may lead to deficiencies. While the dentist is injecting, the chairside assistant fills the impression tray with heavy-bodied material and the tray is seated until the stops come into contact with the teeth. It is held in position until the material has completely set. It is most important that the cavity should remain dry until the tray is fully seated. Cotton-wool rolls should not be accidentally trapped

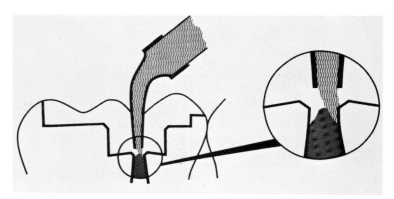

Fig. 9.20 Technique of injecting impression material into adjacent Class II cavities, with an enlarged view of the gingival area.

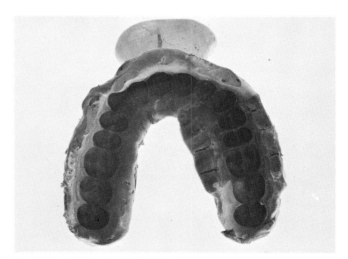

Fig. 9.21 Completed polysulphide rubber impression in a special tray. Note the handle of the tray.

under its margins. In the lower arch the suction tube must be removed immediately before placing in the tray. The setting should be timed accurately and, after the appropriate interval, the tray is withdrawn along the axis of the preparation with a sharp pull. The impression is washed, dried with compressed air and inspected in good light (Fig. 9.21). A good impression should have the following features:

- The material must have flowed into all the internal parts of the cavity and into the whole of the gingival sulcus adjacent to the margins of the preparations.
- It must give sharp reproduction of details.
- There should be no filling defects.
- The impression material should be firmly attached to the tray.

Where extensive undercuts, such as bridge pontics and large interdental spaces, are present, they should be temporarily occluded with wax before taking the impression to avoid tearing the material. For taking an impression of pin-holes, made for example with a 0.6 mm diameter twist drill, a plastic pin, slightly smaller in diameter, is seated in the hole before taking the impression. The pin has a flat head so that it withdraws as part of the impression. Subsequently, an iridio-platinum pin is substituted for it and incorporated in the wax pattern and finished casting.

Finally, a silicone or alginate impression of the opposing arch is obtained.

OCCLUSAL RECORDS

Recording the relationships of upper and lower teeth during functional movements of the mandible, and reproducing these on an articulator for the construction of indirect restorations in the laboratory has proved to be very difficult. A number of complex fully adjustable articulators have been developed for full arch reconstruction work but where a smaller number of teeth are being restored simpler techniques are used. These will often require some slight adjustment to the occlusal surface of the restoration in the patient's mouth.

Where a moderate number of teeth are being restored it is desirable to mount the models on a semi-adjustable articulator and, although it is beyond the scope of this text to describe the technique in detail, some indication of the methods will be given. It is necessary to record centric relation, that is the position of the mandible in which the condyles are guided into the uppermost and rearmost position. In this position the mandible rotates with a simple hinge movement around an axis known as the terminal hinge axis. In addition, the clinician must use a face bow to record the relationship of the upper arch to the glenoid fossae on the base of the skull. He must record the protruded position of the mandible and possibly the right and left side working positions. With this information the models are mounted on the articulator

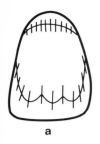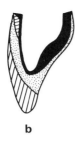

a   b

Fig. 9.22 Aesthetic build up of porcelain jacket crown. (*a*) sketch for laboratory technician; the curved lines gingivally and incisally indicate the junctions between the gingival and body dentine and body dentine and incisal enamel; the vertical straight lines indicate the gradation from one shade to another; (*b*) bucco-lingual cross-section showing the aluminous core (black); body dentine (stippled); gingival dentine (horizontal lines); and incisal enamel (vertical lines).

and the condylar paths adjusted to simulate functional movements in the patient.

For restoring one or two teeth it is often sufficient to mount the moveable die model and the opposing arch model on an average path articulator. Often the models can be correctly articulated without any occlusal record, but unless the dentist has inspected the occlusion in the mouth and is confident that it can be reproduced in the laboratory, a record of centric occlusion should be made. The technique of having the patient occlude on a piece of soft wax often introduces errors since the teeth may not reach centric occlusion and may be deflected. It is better to take right and left buccal records by placing the teeth in centric occlusion and pressing a mix of silicone putty against the buccal surfaces of the teeth until it has set. Some dentists dispense with an articulator and rely on the technician to observe wear facets and simulate jaw movements on hand-held models.

Where the terminal tooth in the arch has been prepared with full occlusal reduction, and particularly if it is isolated, the *transfer coping* technique may be needed. When the final impression of the prepared tooth has been taken, a model is cast and a thin coping or cap is constructed in a contrasting colour of self-curing acrylic resin in the laboratory. The patient is recalled, the temporary restoration removed and the transfer coping fitted. It should fit the preparation accurately and be clear of the opposing teeth in all occlusal movements. A mix of self-curing acrylic resin is made, and when it has reached the correct consistency it is flowed on to the occlusal surface of the coping and the patient guided into centric occlusion. When set this can be transferred to the laboratory and used for the correct mounting of the models.

REPRODUCING NATURAL TEETH IN DENTAL PORCELAIN

With porcelain or porcelain bonded to metal crowns great care must be taken in recording the aesthetic features of the adjacent and contralateral teeth so that the most natural appearance will be obtained in the crown. The teeth should be examined in good natural light or corrected artificial light. If possible, the technician should also inspect the tooth. The main features noted are colour, translucency and texture. Colour and translucency are the result of a combination of light reflected from the tooth surface, light reflected from the underlying dentine surface and light which has passed through the tooth. The latter is responsible for translucency and, since enamel is much less opaque than dentine, translucency is prominent on the incisal edge and sometimes

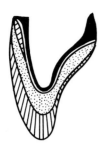

Fig. 9.23 Bucco-lingual cross-section of porcelain bonded to metal crown showing cast metal (black); opaque layer (white); gingival dentine (horizontal lines); body dentine (stippled); and enamel (vertical lines).

mesially and distally. The cervical region is often a different shade from the main body of the tooth.

The appearance must be recorded in detail, preferably with a diagram, so that this can be reproduced in the laboratory (Fig. 9.22). The colours of the different parts are selected by comparison with a shade guide produced by the manufacturer, and the areas and degrees of translucency noted. Examination of the surface texture involves noting the reflectivity of the tooth surface and the contour of the natural grooves and ridges.

The technician will build up the crown in layers of porcelain corresponding to the body dentine, gingival dentine and enamel (Fig. 9.22). Underneath this the porcelain crown will have porcelain core with a high alumina content and the porcelain bonded to metal crown will have a layer of opaque porcelain covering the metal framework (Fig. 9.23). The technician will reproduce the shading translucency and contour of the tooth together with the surface texture, the correct degree of glaze and any permanent intrinsic staining of the enamel and dentine.

COMMUNICATION WITH THE LABORATORY

This is crucially important; poor communication has been the cause of many unsatisfactory restorations when the technician has not been clear in his mind what the clinician required. Where the technician is on the premises he should be involved in planning the restoration and in taking the shade. In any case, all the information the technician requires should be clearly recorded.

It is essential to use a standard form on which is noted the following information:

Patient's name and number; name of clinician; name of technician; date of next appointment; details of work required, including the tooth to be restored, the type of restoration and the material to be used, the stage to which the technician must proceed, for example try-in of metal work, and details of the extent of metal and porcelain coverage in the case of porcelain bonded to metal crown.

PREPARATION OF WORKING MODELS

The full-arch impression will have been checked at the chairside to ensure that it is satisfactory. Unless the impression can be plated with metal it is convenient to pour several sets of dies from the same impression to overcome the risk of abrading these during working.

- Removable die model (Fig. 9.24b). This is the first model cast from the impression and is used for constructing the wax pattern or building up the crown. The use of a dowel pin allows the die to be readily removed from, and replaced precisely in, the model.
- One-piece localisation model (Fig. 9.24c). This is used for getting the contact relationships.
- For metal work it is useful to pour-up a third set of polishing dies, since any damage incurred during finishing and polishing will be confined to these and will leave the original dies intact for checking the finished work or remaking it in the case of a technical error.

The opposing arch impression is cast in dental stone.

LABORATORY TECHNIQUES

A full description of the construction of cast metal and porcelain restorations is outside the scope of this book and the reader is referred to a manual of laboratory procedures.

CHECKING WORK RECEIVED FROM THE LABORATORY

The completed work should be assessed when it has been received from the laboratory. First the models and dies should be inspected carefully, without the work in position, to ensure that they have not been rubbed or abraded, and the occlusion should be inspected. Next the fitting surface of the restoration should be examined to ascertain that it has reproduced the detail of the preparation in reverse and that the technician has not had to grind this surface. The die is removed from the model, the restoration seated on it and the retention and marginal fit assessed. The restoration and die are now reseated in the model and the contacts with the adjacent teeth checked. Finally, the opposing model is brought into occlusion and this is checked. A strip of thin metal foil placed between opposing teeth will confirm that the restoration is in contact and that the remaining teeth in the segment are not out of occlusion. In the case of an aesthetic restoration the shade may be compared with the original shade guide.

FITTING AND FINISHING INLAYS MADE BY
THE DIRECT TECHNIQUE

At the next visit the temporary dressing is removed and the cavity thoroughly cleaned to ensure that all traces of the dressing have

Fig. 9.24 (*and on facing page*)
Laboratory techniques for the
construction of indirect inlays.
(*a*) Part of an impression showing the
preparations. Note the pencil lines
placed by the technician to assist in
positioning the dowel pins.
(*b*) Removable die model with
separate dies on dowel pin. The
occlusal view (*above*) shows one wax
pattern in the course of construction.
(*c*) One-piece model to check contact
areas (*left*). Polishing die (*right*).
(*d*) Completed restorations.

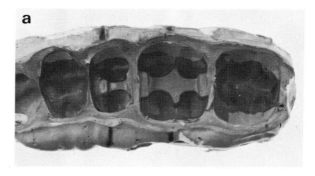

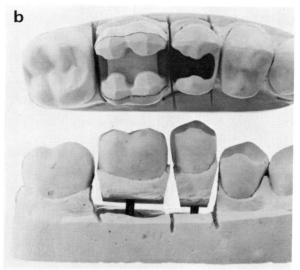

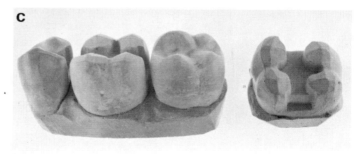

been removed. The inlay, which should still have the sprue
attached, is placed into the cavity and pressed home using firm
finger pressure. If the inlay seats perfectly it is checked carefully
for the following features:

Fig. **9.24** *cont.*

d

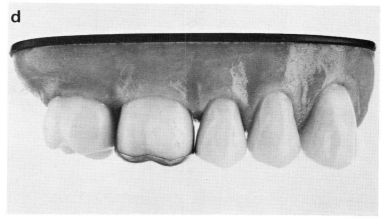

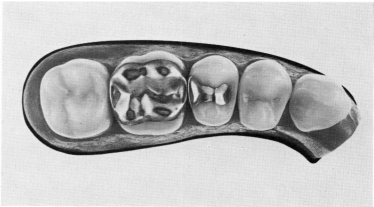

● The marginal adaptation of the whole of the periphery of the inlay should be completely satisfactory, with neither over- nor under-extension.

● The inlay should be sufficiently retentive and some effort should be required to remove it from the cavity.

If the casting does not seat completely it should be removed and the cavity again inspected to ensure that all temporary dressing has been cleared. Likewise the inlay itself should be checked. Usually the fault will be remedied and the inlay made to seat satisfactorily but undue force should not be used to effect this. However, if the inlay still does not seat and there is no indication where the fault lies, the decision should be taken to remake the inlay. On no account should indiscriminate grinding of the fitting surface be undertaken, since this will reduce retention; nor should much time be spent in attempting to get it to fit, since this is usually wasted or leads to an unsatisfactory restoration. Before taking a new impression the cavity should be re-checked to ensure that all parts are withdrawable.

When the inlay is fitting satisfactorily, the sprue should be removed with a fine fissure bur as close to the surface as possible. Finishing and polishing of a direct inlay outside the mouth should be confined to the central areas of the surface and should avoid the peripheral one or two millimetres, otherwise the margins may be damaged; the marginal areas should be finished only on the tooth.

FITTING AND FINISHING RESTORATIONS MADE BY THE INDIRECT TECHNIQUE

At the next visit, using local anaesthesia if necessary, the temporary restoration is removed and the preparation thoroughly cleaned to ensure that all traces of the temporary cement have been cleared away. If the occlusion is involved it must be re-examined at this stage so that the relationship with the opposing teeth before the restoration is seated can be compared with that after seating. In the case of small inlays, such as Class I or Class V, it may be wise to leave the sprue in position to act as a handle until the fit has been checked.

The restoration is placed on the preparation and pressed home using firm finger pressure. If it seats perfectly it is carefully checked for the following features:

- Satisfactory fit around the whole of the periphery with neither over- nor under-extension.
- Adequate retention so that some effort is required to remove it from the preparation. This is particularly important in the case of an inlay.
- Contacts with the adjacent teeth, and contact areas and embrasures which reproduce those found in a normal dentition.
- Correctly contoured buccal and lingual surfaces. Over-contouring should be avoided.
- Correct occlusion. In the case of posterior teeth, when the patient closes in centric occlusion or centric relation, the supporting cusps should be in contact with their opposing fossae, both in the restoration and in the other teeth in the segment. When the mandible moves into a working side relationship the restoration and the other teeth in the segment should slide freely in contact with the cusp slopes of the opposing teeth to the point where cusp-to-cusp contact is reached—group function. An exception is

made in the case of a canine-protected occlusion. In non-working side slide there should be no contact between the restoration and the opposing teeth. As the mandible slides into protrusion the restoration and the neighbouring teeth should slide freely, in contact and without any interference, or move out of contact entirely.

In the case of anterior teeth the restoration and the remaining teeth in the segment should be in contact in centric occlusion and should contact in protrusive slide without any interference.

● Good appearance. In the case of a porcelain or porcelain bonded to metal crown the shades, translucency, intrinsic markings, general form and surface contour should be in harmony with the adjacent and contralateral teeth.

If the restoration fulfils all these requirements it is deemed to be satisfactory and is ready to be cemented. Often some adjustment must be made, but this should be relatively small. If it does not seat completely the contacts with the adjacent teeth should be examined and, if over-contoured, should be reduced until it does seat. Articulating film placed between the restoration and the adjacent tooth will help to locate the spot to be ground. If there is still difficulty the cavity should again be checked to ensure that no temporary cement remains, and the fitting surface of the metal examined for any shiny areas which may indicate a high spot needing reduction. Indicator wax may be helpful. If there is still difficulty it may be better to consider remaking the restoration; certainly it is wise not to spend too much time indiscriminately grinding the fitting surface since this often leads to an unsatisfactory fit and a waste of time. Before re-taking the impression the preparation should again be inspected, especially to make sure that no undercuts are present.

When the restoration is seating satisfactorily the patient may be asked to bite on a piece of soft wood to help seat it as fully as possible, although not with a porcelain jacket crown. At this stage the use of local anaesthesia may disturb the patient's sensation in judging the occlusion and where possible it is better to avoid it. The mandible should be guided into centric occlusion using coloured articulating film between the teeth so as to produce a mark on the area which is high. In the case of metal surfaces this mark is more easily seen if the surface has not been polished or if it has been sandblasted. The restoration is reduced until the supporting cusps meet the corresponding fossae of the opposing teeth to the same extent as the remaining teeth in the segment, with no tendency for the mandible to be displaced. Next, the

173   *Inlays and crowns*

working side movement is checked and adjusted until there is no interference and a free slide is possible. This usually involves the lingual slopes of the upper buccal cusps or the buccal slopes of the lower lingual cusps. Clearly, it is the restoration which should be reduced if the occlusion has been satisfactorily balanced before the start of treatment. In non-working side movements any contact with the opposing teeth is undesirable and the restoration should be reduced accordingly. This usually involves the lingual slopes of the lower buccal cusps or the buccal slopes of the upper lingual cusps. Finally, it should be balanced in protrusive slide which usually involves distal-facing slopes of upper teeth or mesial-facing slopes of lower teeth.

After the occlusion has been adjusted the restoration must be removed from the mouth, smoothed with finishing stones and discs and polished. The occlusal surface may be sand-blasted so that any occlusal interferences will be clearly visible at the next appointment, when the final adjusting and finishing will be done. The restoration is now ready to be cemented.

CEMENTATION

Prior to cementation the restoration should be cleaned and dried and the preparation isolated and dried. Cementing medium is mixed to the consistency recommended by the manufacturer and applied rapidly in a thin layer to the whole of the fitting surface.

It is carried to the mouth, seated in position, pressed home firmly under finger pressure and held until the initial set of the cement has taken place. Some operators use a piece of soft wood positioned between the clenched teeth to press the restoration fully home, but this can allow the restoration to tilt and so must be employed with care. After the cement has set it is important to remove all excess. Buccally and lingually a probe or excavator is useful for this but care must be taken not to spoil the polish. Approximally, dental floss in which a knot has been tied is effective in removing any remaining cement. Particular care must be taken, if polycarboxylate cement is used, to remove the excess, either before it becomes rubbery or after it has set. Attempts to remove it at the rubbery stage may result in dragging some of the cement from between the fitting surfaces. If desired the margins may be varnished to protect the newly set cement from saliva.

At the next visit the occlusion should be re-checked and adjusted if necessary. Floss should be used interdentally to ensure that the patient has no difficulty in cleaning this area. Restorations made by the direct method may need some adjustment of the

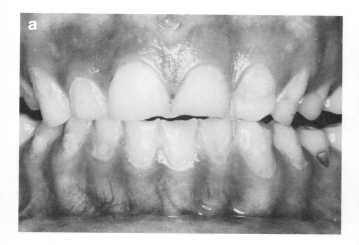

a

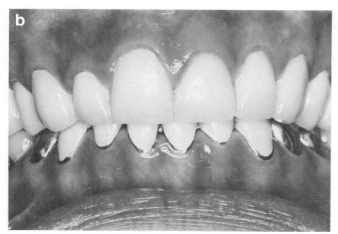

b

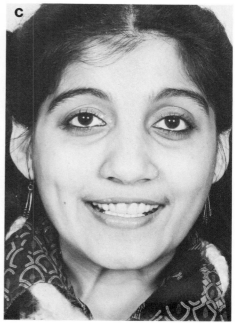

c

Fig. 9.25a The dentition of a 21 year old woman, which is badly affected by tooth surface loss, mainly due to erosion, and which has a number of unsatisfactory Class V restorations.

Fig. 9.25b The same dentition after restoration. All the upper teeth and the lower incisors and canines have been restored by porcelain bonded to metal crowns. In the lower anterior teeth the position of the lip allowed the use of a metal-to-tooth finish labially without detriment to the appearance. Three lower premolar teeth have been restored by full veneer gold crowns.

Fig. 9.25c The patient after treatment.

margins so that these are flush with the adjacent tooth surface. In Fig. 9.25 are shown the pre-operative and post-operative photographs of a girl whose mutilated dentition was restored by crowns.

CAST RESTORATIONS AS RETAINERS FOR PARTIAL DENTURES

The preparation of a mouth for the reception of partial dentures may involve some re-shaping of the natural teeth to provide parallel guiding planes, seats for occlusal rests, provision of space for clasp arms to pass across the occlusal surface and provision of the correct degree of undercut for the retentive arms of clasps. The design for the partial denture must be completed before any

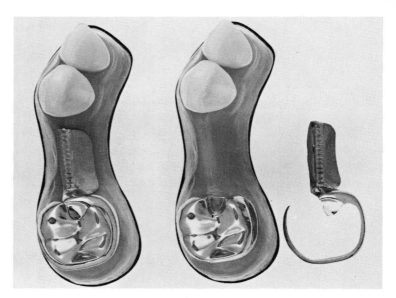

Fig. 9.26 Full cast crown designed to receive the clasp of a partial denture. (*Left*) clasp in position; (*right*) clasp and crown separated. Note the seat for the occlusal rest and the ledge for the bracing part of the clasp. The correct degree of undercut is built into the buccal surface to provide retention.

treatment of a permanent nature is commenced so that the precise sites of rest seats, parallel guiding planes and clasps are established. It frequently happens that a tooth planned for use as an abutment either has a restoration or requires to be restored and in these cases the restoration must be designed in such a way that it can accommodate the partial denture (Green & Bates 1981). For example, a Class II restoration designed to support an occlusal rest will require to have adequate thickness to accommodate the rest and still have sufficient strength.

Sometimes it is preferable to have a full veneer gold or porcelain bonded to gold crown into which the required contours are built at the wax pattern stage, as this can permit a precise re-shaping of the tooth (Fig. 9.26). The preparation for the crown must include sufficient tooth removal to allow for adequate thickness of crown and the extension of the denture into it. A full arch model with removable precision dies is constructed and surveyed prior to mounting on an articulator. During the preparation of the wax pattern parallel guiding planes can be provided by contouring on a surveyor. The base of the guiding planes forms a shoulder which acts as a rest and supports the bracing arm. At the same time the contour necessary to provide retention for the retentive clasp arm is built on to the pattern. Several such precision-fitting crowns can greatly increase the stability and retention of a partial denture.

A further extension of the principle is the incorporation of prefabricated precision attachments into the crown which can provide excellent retention for partial dentures, incorporating a stress-breaking action where required and, by the elimination of clasps, improving aesthetics.

References and further reading

CHRISTENSON G.J. (1966) *J. prosth. Dent.* **16,** 297–305.
GREEN R.M. & BATES J.F. (1981) *Dent. Update*, **8,** 263–266.
GRIEVE A.R. & GLYN JONES J.C. (1981) *Brit. dent. J.* **151,** 331–334.
LOREY R.E. & MYERS G.E. (1968) *J. Amer. dent. Ass.* **76,** 568–572.
SHILLINGBURG H.T., HOBO S. & WHITSETT L.D. (1981) *Fundamentals of Fixed Prosthodontics.* 2nd ed. Quintessence, Chicago.
SMITH B.G.N. (1970) *J. prosth. Dent.* **23,** 187–198.
STANANOUGHT D. (1975) *Laboratory Procedures for Inlays, Crowns and Bridges.* Blackwell Scientific Publications, Oxford.

Chapter 10
Organisation and working methods

One of the aims of a dental student must be to develop skill in the practice of conservative dentistry. This involves not only the ability to achieve a desired objective, but also its achievement in the minimum of time and with the minimum of effort. Observation of a highly skilled worker, whether manual or otherwise, will show that he appears to work in a relaxed and purposeful manner, without rushing and without unnecessary movements or activities; at the same time he achieves a successful end-result. The dental student must strive towards this although it may take some years before he becomes highly skilled. His skill will be of value to his patients since they will not only receive better treatment but will receive it in a shorter time, in more relaxed surroundings and they are more likely to be seen punctually; it will help to build the patient's confidence in him. The dentist who is tense and rushing cannot expect his patients to be relaxed and cannot expect to have the best possible relationship with them. Working in a relaxed manner should help the dentist to be less affected by stress and it is obviously desirable for him to avoid spending unnecessary time on treatment, provided that a good standard of work is achieved.

The student should realise from the beginning of his training the importance of organising his work. It is not satisfactory for him to learn to work in a disorganised manner and then to try to impose a pattern of organisation upon it. It is better for him to learn techniques and organisation together from the beginning of his course. He should appreciate that, under modern conditions of practice, a high degree of efficiency is essential for the dentist who wishes to run an economically successful practice and maintain good standards.

Ergonomics

It is only comparatively recently that the principles of efficient working, developed in industry, have been applied to dentistry. This has resulted in extensive re-thinking of operating methods used in dentistry with the result that the modern dentist sits while he is operating, with his patient in a near-horizontal position. At the same time the dental manufacturer has made considerable changes in the design of his equipment so that it is now possible to obtain equipment which facilitates relaxed and efficient working.

Ergonomics can be defined as the economic use of human endeavour with adjustment of the working requirements to physical and psychological conditions. When applied to dentistry its objectives are to make it possible for the dentist, helped by his assistant, to deliver the maximum quantity of high quality dental care to the maximum number of people with reasonable comfort and with the minimum of stress.

BASIC PRINCIPLES OF ERGONOMICS

The basic principles of ergonomics are as follows:

- *Eliminate* all unnecessary items of equipment, instruments, steps in procedures and movements.
- *Combine* the functions of two or more instruments or items of equipment or steps in a procedure. Examples are the triple syringe which can produce either a water jet, an air jet or an air and water spray; double-ended instruments; dual-purpose burs such as the dome-ended fissure bur; and the spray attachment on handpieces which avoids the necessity for a dental assistant to operate a separate water spray.
- *Re-arrange* items of equipment, steps in procedures, scheduling of patients so as to take better advantage of available time and space. For example, during cavity preparations it may not be advisable to carry out the stages of cavity preparation always in the same order, sometimes it may be more efficient to change the order. The repositioning of an item of equipment in the surgery may enable it to be more readily reached by the assistant or dentist.
- *Simplify* equipment and treatment procedures so as to enable work to be carried out more efficiently and reduce the risk of breakdown or mishap.

The application of these principles should enable the operator gradually to develop an efficient working technique. The principles impress on him the need to simplify and reduce the number of body movements and the distance moved. Instruments should be located as conveniently as possible for the person who has to use them, either the assistant or the dentist. Several functions of instruments may be combined and unnecessary instruments should be eliminated.

This commences with the formulation of a treatment plan which should be clearly set out in writing and should indicate the sequence of items of treatment.

In making an appointment it is essential for the dentist to inform the chairside assistant precisely which procedures are to be carried out during the proposed visit so that sufficient time can be allowed and so that the appropriate instruments and materials can be available. Where more complex treatment is involved several appointments may need to be arranged at appropriate intervals.

Failure to make a correct diagnosis may lead to inefficiency; for example, if several occlusal restorations are planned and, through faulty diagnosis, associated approximal cavities are not discovered until treatment has commenced, some degree of disorganisation will result. Bitewing radiographs, together with careful clinical examination, should enable an accurate diagnosis of approximal caries to be made and some assessment of the extent of the carious lesions. In the same way, failure to recognise that a patient is abnormally apprehensive may lead to a dentist planning to carry out too much work during an appointment.

Failure to plan the sequence of treatment correctly may also lead to inefficiency. If, for example, a detailed plan of a partial denture is not made before abutment teeth are restored then it may prove difficult and time-consuming to modify the restorations to provide rest seats, parallel guiding planes and retention for clasps.

During the early part of his training the dental student will tend to think in terms of restoring individual teeth, but with experience he should begin to think of preparing and restoring several cavities in the same quadrant. This is possible with high-speed cutting methods and the help of a surgery assistant. Quadrant dentistry may allow one administration of local anaesthetic to be used for a number of teeth, may allow the operator to prepare several cavities simultaneously, to line and fill these at the same visit or to take a single impression of several preparations. Adjacent approximal cavities should in general be prepared simultaneously rather than one being restored before the other is commenced, but it is not wise to restore adjacent teeth at one sitting else the contacts may not be satisfactory.

It is best to avoid unnecessary complications in treatment since the simpler the operation, the greater the chance of success. Thus a full veneer gold crown may be preferable to a complex inlay. On the other hand, it is foolish to ignore problems in the hope that they will disappear. They should be dealt with effectively. For

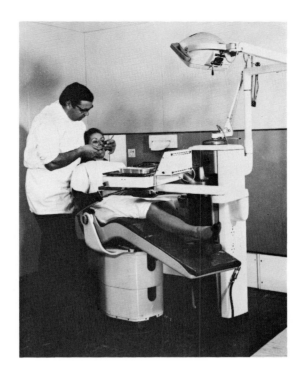

example, if gingival haemorrhage occurs during cavity preparation it should be controlled as soon as possible.

On account of the usual subdivision of dental teaching into disciplines students may fail to consider the possibility of combining two types of treatment on one visit. Sometimes one tooth may be restored and another extracted, possibly within the same area of anaesthesia.

Organisation within the working area

OPERATING POSITIONS

The operating positions used in dentistry for many years were based primarily on the concept that the patient should first be positioned sitting comfortably in a chair with only a slight backwards tilt. The dentist then stood at the right side of the chair and operated (Fig. 10.1). Attempts on his part to sit while operating in order to rest his legs were not entirely successful since the high stool required was uncomfortable and somewhat unstable. Either sitting or standing the dentist frequently had to

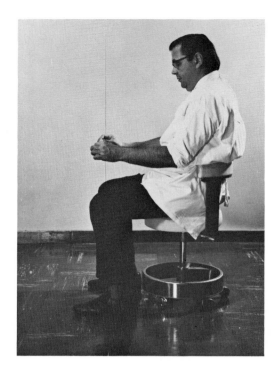

stoop and to twist his body. In addition the standing dentist often placed his weight largely on his right leg while his left foot operated the speed control for the handpiece.

Modern methods for the treatment of patients, using the low-seated position, evolved with the realisation that the conventional methods involved the dentist in unnecessary fatigue and postural difficulties. A reappraisal of the problem commenced by first placing the dentist comfortably seated on an operating stool (Fig. 10.2) and then attempting to position the patient (Figs 10.3 and 10.4), assistant and equipment (Fig. 10.5) so that the dentist could operate with good posture and the minimum of fatigue while at the same time maintaining the patient's comfort. The advent of the air turbine, with its spray which made the use of the dental mirror difficult, did much to stimulate dentists to think about evolving a position where direct vision was possible without the necessity of adopting a poor posture.

The right-handed dentist usually sits at 11 o'clock (Fig. 10.6) but may choose to adopt any position between 12 o'clock and 8 o'clock. The chairside assistant is seated at about 4 or 5 o'clock, at a slightly higher level than the dentist, so that she can see clearly

Fig. 10.3 The patient reclines on a
low-line chair in a horizontal position
while the dentist works from behind.

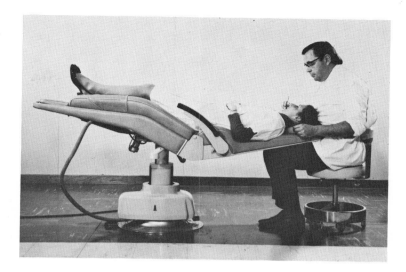

Fig. 10.4 The dentist is working from
the side. The chair is articulated and
can be moved to and from the seated
position by an automatic control. The
backrest is thin so that the knees of
the dentist can be accommodated.

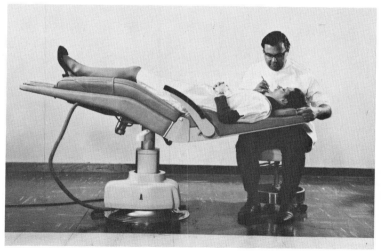

into the mouth. The chair is positioned at an angle of about 15°
elevation of the head.

There are disadvantages in the use of the low-seated technique
and certain contra-indications. It increases the risk of a patient
inhaling or ingesting any small objects which are accidentally
dropped in the mouth, such as inlays, dentine pins, small
endodontic instruments and fragments of amalgam. Protection
should be used when any of these are introduced into the mouth.
Rubber dam is the best protection. The butterfly sponge (Figs.
10.7 and 10.8) is valuable, particularly for treatment under

183   *Organisation and working methods*

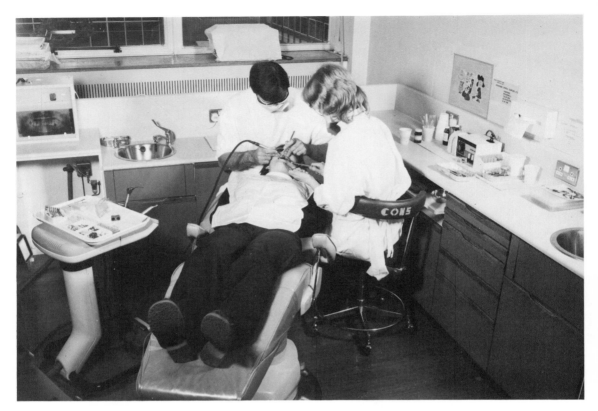

Fig. 10.5 The assistant, positioned at 4 o'clock, joins the dentist and the patient. The dental unit is convenient to the dentist's right hand, there is a working surface or writing area behind him and the wash basin and X-ray viewer are alongside. The assistant has a triple syringe, suction tubes and spitting funnel built into the cabinetry near her right hand (out of sight) and a slide-out shelf for the hand instruments. The cabinetry provides her with a work surface for preparation of filling materials, cupboards and drawers for storage and a wash basin.

sedation, and a napkin can be useful if correctly placed (Fig. 10.9). Latch-type burs should be firmly locked in the handpiece before use.

There is also a risk of causing eye damage to a reclining patient if an instrument being passed across the face is accidentally dropped. Instruments should never be passed or exchanged above a patient's face and as a further precaution protective spectacles should be provided. If these are coloured they will also shield the eyes from glare. Some patients, particularly the old and very apprehensive, dislike the fully horizontal position. In others it may be contra-indicated on medical grounds such as nasal obstruction, hiatus hernia, Ménière's disease and those taking anti-hypertensive drugs.

Operating on Lower teeth

The chair is usually positioned at about 15° to the horizontal with the headrest tilted slightly forward so that the occlusal plane of the

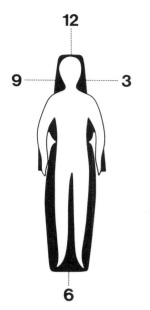

Fig. 10.6 Clock-face notation used to describe the relationship of personnel and equipment to the patient's mouth.

lower teeth is roughly horizontal (Fig. 10.10). The dentist operates from the 11 o'clock position, or sometimes from 8 o'clock.

Lower right segment   The dentist operates using a finger rest on the adjacent teeth. When he is cutting with the high-speed handpiece, the assistant holds the suction tube between the field of operation and the tongue so that spray is removed and the tongue is protected from accidental damage (Fig. 10.11). Alternatively, a flanged suction tube may be held in position by the patient.

Lower anterior segment   The dentist operates from the 11 o'clock position using a finger rest on the lower right teeth. The assistant may retract the lip with one hand and with the other she holds the suction tube lingual to the teeth to collect spray and protect the tongue.

Lower left segment   The dentist uses the anterior teeth as a finger rest. The assistant holds the suction tube in the buccal sulcus and the patient holds a flanged suction tube between the tongue and the field of operation, mainly to act as a tongue guard (Fig. 10.12).

Operating on Upper teeth

For upper teeth the chair should be about 15° to the horizontal with the headrest tilted back so that the upper occlusal plane is nearly vertical (Fig. 10.10). Operating is normally carried out from the 11 o'clock approach using mirror vision and with the light beam nearly vertical. When cutting with a spray, direct vision from the 9 o'clock position is sometimes useful, with light coming in from the front at about 45°.

Upper left quadrant

The dentist obtains a finger rest anteriorly. The assistant may retract the cheek with a finger of the right hand and with the other hand she positions the suction tube in the buccal sulcus (Fig. 10.13).

Upper anterior segment

The dentist operates on the labial aspect using direct vision with a finger rest in the upper right quadrant. The assistant holds the suction tube below, that is lingual to, the area of operation. When

Fig. 10.7 Butterfly sponge.

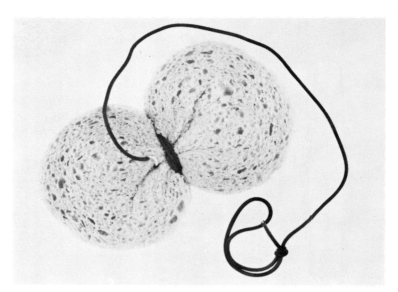

Fig. 10.8 The butterfly sponge, shown in position for operating on the upper left quadrant, will effectively prevent the passage of foreign bodies into the pharynx. Only half of the sponge is in the mouth.

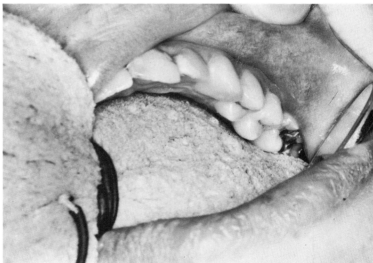

operating from the lingual approach, the mirror is used; any spray reaching the mirror can be cleared by the assistant directing a steady stream of air over its surface and holding the suction tube close to it.

Upper right quadrant

This is treated in a similar manner to the upper anterior segment except that there may not be room for more than one rest finger.

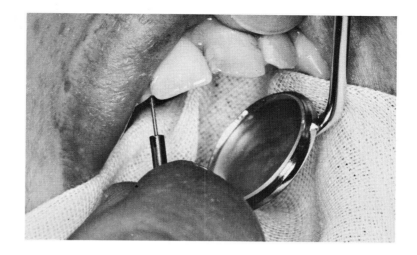

Fig. 10.9 A dental napkin, carefully positioned, will help to prevent the passage of a foreign body.

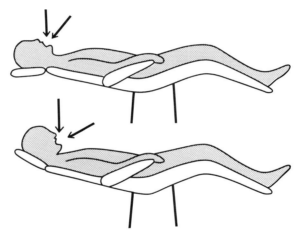

Fig. 10.10 Positions of the patient for operating on upper teeth (*above*) and lower teeth (*below*). In each case the chair back should be about 15° to the horizontal but for upper teeth the headrest should be tilted slightly backwards and for lower teeth, slightly forwards. The beam of light should be adjusted carefully depending on whether direct or mirror vision is being used.

WORK AREAS

These are areas which the dentist and assistant can reach without any inconvenience while they are seated in the normal operating positions.

Reference to Figs 10.14 and 10.15 will show that the dentist, seated at 9 o'clock and 12 o'clock and the assistant seated at 4 o'clock have primary work areas which can be reached by forearm movement alone and secondary work areas which can be reached by full arm movement. The patient's mouth should be within the primary work areas of the dentist and the assistant. Within the primary or secondary work area of the dentist, either on his right

Fig. 10.11 Operating on the lower right quadrant. The assistant holds the suction tube between the tongue and the teeth and retracts the lip.

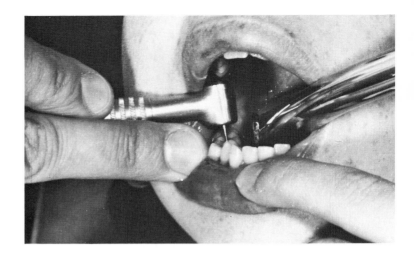

Fig. 10.12 Operating on the lower left quadrant. The assistant holds a suction tube in the buccal sulcus.

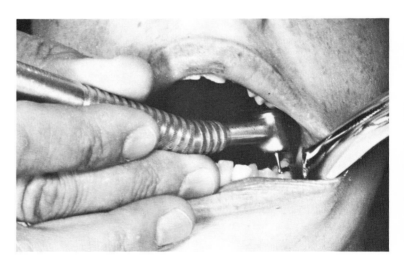

or perhaps in front of him, should be positioned the high-speed and low-speed handpieces and a triple syringe.

Within the primary or secondary work area of the assistant should be the tray of instruments, the high-volume suction tubes, a second triple syringe and an area for storage and mixing of materials. The general principle is that frequently used items of equipment and materials should be positioned within easy reach and without the need for the assistant to turn; less frequently used items should be further away and accessible to the assistant if she rotates on her stool.

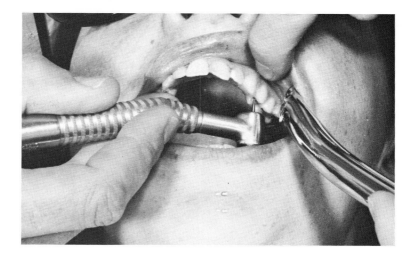

Fig. 10.13 Operating on the upper left quadrant using direct vision. The assistant holds the suction tube and retracts the lip.

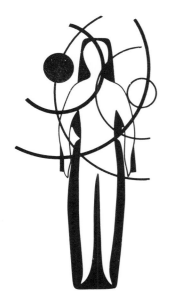

Fig. 10.14 Work areas. The dentist (*black circle*) working at the 9 o'clock position can reach the inner arc (*heavy line*) with forearm movements and the outer arc with full arm movements. The assistant (*white circle*), seated at the 4 o'clock position, can reach the inner and outer arcs with forearm and arm movements respectively.

HAND INSTRUMENTS

From an ergonomic view point it is highly desirable to have instruments in kits. In this way the dentist can have the instruments required for any operation in a set order in the tray. It will simplify the finding of a particular instrument and, if the tray is properly designed, the instrument can be readily grasped and put into use (Fig. 10.16). Instruments can be marked with strips of adhesive tape which will resist sterilisation, using different colours to indicate different kits and different levels to show the position each instrument occupies in the tray. Trays can be sterilised and stored near the chairside ready for use; this arrangement saves time when transferring from one patient to another. Sterilised and used instruments should never be mixed together and must have separate storage areas.

WORKING WITH THE DENTAL SURGERY ASSISTANT

When working with a dental surgery assistant the student or dentist should, as far as possible, standardise procedures since variations in his operating technique will make it more difficult for the assistant to anticipate his needs. For the same reason, he should keep to a minimum the number of instruments used and try to develop a clear and efficient pattern of work.

The student should not expect the impossible from his assistant. It is his responsibility to make sure that she understands clearly what duties she is expected to carry out. Before the patient arrives, she should be able to consult the appointment book or case

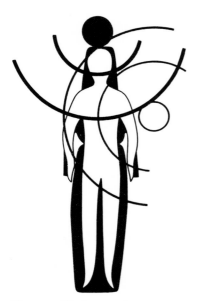

Fig. 10.15 Work areas, showing the forearm and arm reach of the dentist (*black circle*), working at 12 o'clock, and assistant (*white circle*).

notes and know what procedure is planned, the time allocated and any special instruments or equipment required.

The student should not expect to be proficient at working with an assistant at first. It is best for him to attempt simple procedures with her help, until these can be carried out satisfactorily, before trying more advanced procedures. He should always treat his assistant politely, compliment her when she does well, thank her at the end of each session for her help, and occasionally tell her tactfully how she can improve, but never in front of the patient. He should encourage her to make suggestions for the improvement of the practice, recognise her as the essential member of the team she is, and work to achieve a good relationship with her. Most dental schools now give training in this important aspect of dentistry.

As far as possible, the assistant should do everything that the dentist need not do himself. She is responsible for preparing the surgery and having available all the equipment and materials needed. She will make the patient comfortable in the chair and fit the protective covering. The dentist himself will usually position the chair to suit the operation while the assistant prepares the surface anaesthetic and the syringe for injection of local anaesthetic. During the use of the air turbine the assistant will control the high-volume suction tube and retract the soft tissues (Fig. 10.17). She will automatically air-dry the cavity when the dentist removes his handpiece, so that he can inspect it. During low-speed cutting she will hold the triple syringe and suction tube ready to spray out, aspirate and dry the cavity for the dentist to inspect. She will pass any hand instruments which he requires; he may have to ask for these but if a standardised working technique is established she will generally know which instrument is required next. The dentist should extend his hand in such a way that she can read whether he wishes to use the pen grasp or the palm and thumb grasp and will position the instrument accordingly in his hand so that no adjustment is required before use. She may even be able to anticipate which end of the instrument he will use. The passing and receiving of instruments is simple if the assistant has both hands available (Fig. 10.18) but if one hand is occupied she will have to learn to receive a used instrument and pass a fresh instrument with one hand (Fig. 10.19). Instruments should never be passed over the patient's face in case one is accidentally dropped. Changing burs may be done either by the assistant or by the dentist.

After completion of the cavity, and while the dentist is isolating it, the assistant should prepare the lining material and hold it close

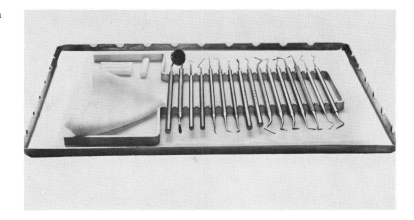

Fig. 10.16 Kit of hand instruments in a rack. The instruments should always be placed in the same sequence. Note that they may be readily grasped by the dentist in the centre of the handle, or by the assistant at the end of the handle.

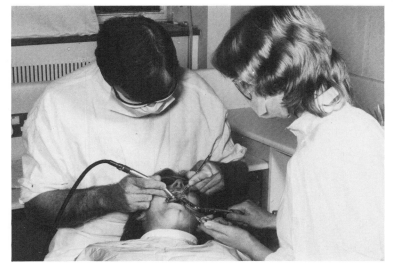

Fig. 10.17 Four-handed dentistry. The dentist, using indirect vision with the aid of a mirror, is preparing a cavity with the air turbine handpiece while the dental surgery assistant uses the suction tube to remove the coolant after use. Her left hand holds the triple syringe ready to dry the cavity immediately the handpiece is removed from the mouth.

to the patient's mouth, at the same time handing the dentist the instrument required for the insertion. The assistant should prepare the matrix, mix the permanent filling material, and pass any instruments necessary for its insertion and carving. With accessible cavities she can place amalgam into the cavity ready for the dentist to condense; this will avoid an unnecessary exchange of instruments. At the end of treatment she will help to tidy up the patient's face, remove the protective covering and assist the patient from the chair.

A good chairside assistant will develop the ability to anticipate the dentist's actions and prepare for them. It is worth emphasising that techniques for increased efficiency do not necessarily mean

191   *Organisation and working methods*

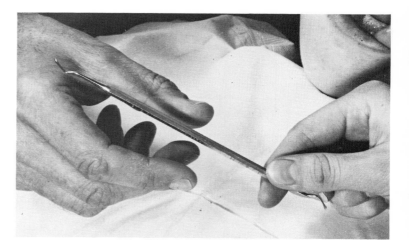

Fig. 10.18 Instrument transfer. The assistant (*on right*) holds the instrument near its end and places it in the dentist's hand which is positioned to indicate that he will use the pen grasp. Note that this transfer does not take place above the patient's face.

that the dentist becomes overworked or the patient is treated impersonally. Certainly this may happen, but not if the dentist is correctly orientated towards the welfare of his patients and towards his own health. Efficient working methods should give the dentist more time to develop good relationships with his patients.

Surgery design

A well-planned surgery should fulfil three requirements. It should be functional, that is it should enable all the required types of work to be carried out efficiently. It should not increase apprehension but should if possible assist the patient to relax; pieces of equipment which the patient may find upsetting should be either hidden or inconspicuous. Finally, the surgery layout and equipment should be aesthetically pleasing; very dull and very bright colours should be avoided.

Although it is possible to use a room 2.5 m square as a surgery this is restricting and dimensions of 2.5 m by 3 or 3 m by 3.5 are preferable. If a larger room has to be used then it is wise to separate off the optimum area for the surgery and use the remainder for some other purpose.

As a first stage in surgery design, a dentist must specify the work patterns which he plans to use and the storage areas which will be required in the surgery. Then he can consider the floor plan. A useful aid is to mark out the outline of the room to a scale of say 1 : 10 on a sheet of stiff cardboard. The door and windows should be included and any permanent structures which may affect the design. Outlines of major items of equipment and cabinets are

Fig. 10.19 Single-handed instrument exchange.
(*a*) The assistant receives the excavator between her third and fourth fingers and (*b*) places the tweezers in the dentist's hand ready for use with the pen grasp.

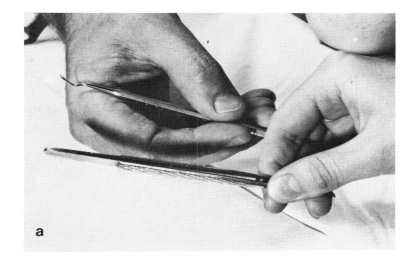

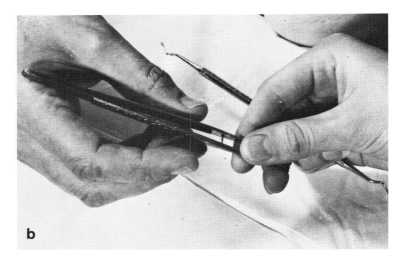

drawn to the same scale on cardboard and cut out; different colours may be used for different types of equipment to give greater contrast. Double-sided adhesive tape is fitted on the back of each piece.

The first step is to position the chair provisionally within the outline of the room. At one time it was necessary to have the chair facing the window so that the dentist might, as far as possible, use natural light both for operating and for checking shades, and so that the patient might look out of the window. However, improved lights and extensive use of the reclining position have made it

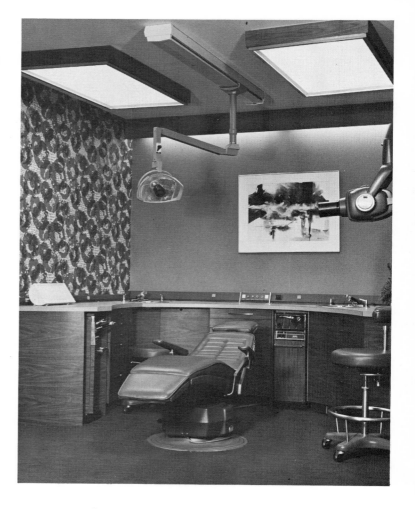

unnecessary for the chair to face the window. Generally, it should be positioned so that the patient may enter without passing through the work area of the chairside assistant. This usually means that it is most convenient for the patient to enter the chair from the 7 or 8 o'clock position and the chair is often placed obliquely so that this position is directly opposite the door. Next, the position from which the dentist will operate for most of the time should be decided. He may, for example, use the 11 o'clock area while the assistant is stationed at 4 o'clock.

On these positions will depend the placing of the dentist's and the assistant's units. A decision must be made as to whether the assistant will be available continuously or occasionally. The dentist's unit should have two handpieces and a triple syringe. The assistant will require a work surface, mobile or fixed, for holding instruments and mixing materials, a triple syringe, and large bore and small bore suction tubes. A spitting funnel will be needed. Both these units should be mobile, mounted either on casters or in a hinged or extending arm, so that they can be moved out of the way when not in use. If only occasional assistance is available the hand instruments will have to be kept in such a position that they can be reached by both dentist and assistant.

Built-in storage units should be arranged so that the assistant can reach them without rising from her stool. Separate sink units are needed for dentist and assistant; that for the assistant must be large and close to her work area. Finally, the chair must be re-positioned so as to give the best relationship to the storage units, the dentist and the assistant. It is now common for surgery equipment to be supplied in modular form so that the individual can select the best designs and the best arrangement for his needs. Fig. 10.20 shows an example of a modern surgery.

Finally, all the common movement patterns which the dentist, assistant and patient will undertake should be envisaged in detail to ensure that no unnecessary or inconvenient movement is involved. Similarly, movement of instruments and equipment to and from the operating area should be considered.

These principles can be extended to include the planning of full practice accommodation including waiting room, office, surgeries and laboratory. Patterns of patient and staff flow should be considered. Thus a complete list of movements of staff and patients during a sample period may be prepared and the paths of movement laid out on a scale plan of the premises using coloured thread or insulated wire. Careful thought should be given to these lines and, in particular, to eliminating unnecessary movements, shortening each line of movement and as far as possible avoiding crossing of routes. A more detailed discussion of surgery design is given elsewhere (Eccles 1977).

OBJECTS OF PRACTICE ORGANISATION

The objects of practice organisation should be:

- To reduce stress and fatigue in the dentist and his assistant.
- To carry out treatment efficiently while maintaining a good standard of work.
- To help the patient feel more relaxed and to provide a better opportunity for developing good relationships with patients.
- To enable the dentist to run a financially successful practice.

Further reading

ECCLES J.D. (1977) *Dental Update* **4,** 275–279.
KILPATRICK H.C. (1974) *Work Simplification in Dental Practice*, 3rd ed. Saunders, Philadelphia.
SCHÖN F. & KIMMEL K. (1968) *Ergonomie in der zahnärtzlichen Praxis.* 'Die Quintessenz', Berlin.

Chapter 11
Control of fluids in the mouth

There are many occasions during conservation treatment and caries prevention when the control of moisture is essential. The introduction of high-speed cutting techniques, with the large volume of water needed for cooling purposes, required a complete re-thinking of the problem of water control resulting in the development of high-volume suction equipment.

Reasons for control

● *Convenience and efficiency*   Moisture control is required for the convenience of the patient and the dentist. Substantial quantities of water in the mouth are unpleasant for the patient and make the work of the dentist difficult. Time is wasted if the patient has to use the spittoon frequently.

● *Visibility*   In the inspection of teeth for the detection of caries or other abnormalities, and in the inspection of cavities during preparation, the presence of water or saliva may distort vision and alter the reflective characteristics of the surface; for example, the matt appearance of early enamel caries may be missed. Haemorrhage from gingival margins may obscure cavities in course of preparation.

● *Best use of materials*   During the insertion of fillings and the cementing of inlays, crowns and bridges, the tooth must be isolated and dried since moisture may interfere with the setting reaction of the materials. It may also prevent the achievement of good marginal adaptation and may reduce the 'adhesion' of the lining, filling or cementing materials. This is particularly the case when etching a tooth surface with acid to provide retention. When taking impressions of prepared teeth, moisture and blood must be excluded. During the insertion of fillings and the taking of impressions near the gingival margins the flow of fluid in this region must be controlled. In preventive measures such as the topical application of fluoride gel or solution or of fissure sealants moisture control is important.

- *Asepsis* Where asepsis is necessary, as in endodontic treatment, the area must be isolated from saliva and respired air.

Methods of control

- Suction—high-volume
            —low-volume
- Absorbents
- Compressed air
- Rubber dam

HIGH-VOLUME SUCTION

For controlling the comparatively large quantity of water where spray cooling is used during high-speed cutting, it is essential to have an aspirating system capable of dealing with high volumes. A suction tube 10.0–12.5 mm internal diameter is held by the surgery assistant in a position to remove as much water as possible, after this has been used to cool the tooth. This tube is connected to the suction equipment by means of a flexible tube of similar diameter and having a smooth internal surface.

Suction equipment High-volume suction can be obtained by means of individual mobile units or a central evacuation system. The mobile unit or aspirator consists of a cabinet containing an electric motor operating a fan with a large bottle for the collection of water and debris. It incorporates an automatic cut-off which operates when the collection bottle is full and involves the inconvenience of emptying the bottle.

The central evacuation system is generally used in clinics or multiple surgeries. It consists of a central vacuum pump connected by wide-bore tubes to a separating chamber or canister in each surgery. The separator is connected by flexible tubes to the suction tubes used in the mouth and contains a filter which separates out solid debris; liquid waste is run off into the drains while the air is passed through the vacuum pump to the outside atmosphere. Such a system is known as a dry-line system to distinguish it from other systems where moisture and air are not separated. Central evacuation systems are best installed during the construction of a clinic. They have the advantage over self-contained units that the emptying of bottles is not required and there is less noise. The separator takes up less space in the surgery than the aspirator and any bacteria which are carried in the air stream are evacuated outside the building and not into the surgery.

Fig. 11.1 Suction tubes. At the top is a wide-bore angled suction tube; below this is a disposable saliva ejector which can be bent to any desired shape; in the centre is a flanged suction tube, valuable in the lower posterior region to limit tongue movements; below this is a right-angled suction tube with bevelled plastic nozzle, and at the bottom is a small-bore curved suction tube.

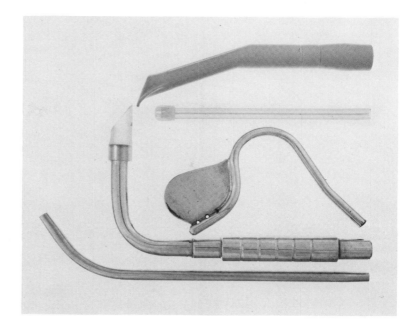

Suction fittings A large variety of tubes are available for high-volume suction; several of these are shown in Fig. 11.1. The most commonly used is a right-angled metal or plastic tube of 10 mm internal diameter having a bevelled end. This is used by the surgery assistant for the collection of spray. A smaller tube of about 6 mm internal diameter is used by the surgery assistant for scavenging particles of filling materials and other solid debris from the mouth. Some tubes incorporate a flange to protect the tongue, and the field of operation, from its unrestrained movements. Small plastic tubes which can be bent to any required shape are used for keeping the mouth free from saliva or small volumes of fluid. The hand spittoon connected to the suction equipment consists of a metal or plastic funnel. This has largely replaced the old type of fixed spittoon bowl flushed with water which is difficult for the reclining patient to reach and occupies valuable space at the chairside.

ABSORBENTS

Absorbent materials such as cotton wool rolls, gauze napkins and absorbent pads, are valuable for short-term control of saliva provided that they are replaced before they become saturated. They should be strategically placed in relation to the salivary

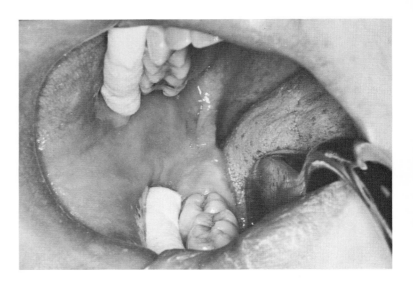

ducts. For isolation of upper posterior teeth a cotton wool roll should be placed opposite the opening of the parotid duct to absorb saliva as it emerges. For isolation of lower posterior teeth a cotton wool roll in the upper buccal sulcus and an additional roll in the lower buccal sulcus should be combined with the use of a suction tube (Fig. 11.2). For isolation of anterior teeth a halved dental napkin twisted into the labial sulcus is valuable (Fig. 11.3). Absorbent pads are manufactured in a number of sizes, generally in a triangular shape with rounded corners to fit into the vestibule opposite the molar teeth (Fig. 11.4). Absorbent material may be used in conjunction with a saliva ejector or a suction tube. Rolls and napkins should be inspected before removal. If they are dry and adherent to the oral mucosa they should be moistened before removal otherwise they may tear away the surface layer of the epithelium resulting in after-pain and ulceration.

Control of fluid from the gingival sulcus may cause difficulties during the insertion of restorations adjacent to the gingival margin. This problem may be overcome by the use of rubber dam, to be described later, or by the use of dry gingival retraction fibre. Retraction fibre may consist of a four-strand cord which can be cut into suitable lengths and if necessary divided into one or more strands according to the depth of the gingival sulcus.

COMPRESSED AIR

Triple syringes, which give the choice of air, air and water spray, or a water jet, are valuable in the control of moisture. After

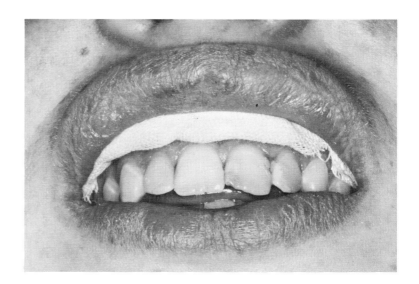

Fig. 11.3 Half-napkin used to isolate upper anterior teeth.

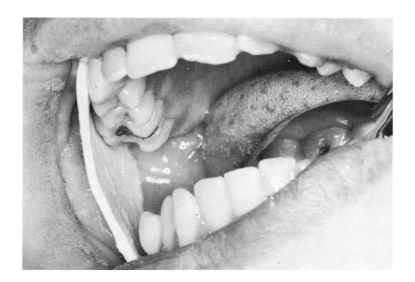

Fig. 11.4 Absorbent pad used in conjunction with a suction tube to isolate posterior teeth.

isolation, the teeth are dried with an air jet and this may be repeated during the treatment as required. There is experimental evidence to indicate that excessive air drying of cavities may lead to some degree of pulpal damage; this should be avoided and only sufficient air used to ensure that the cavity is dry but not dehydrated.

201   *Control of fluids in the mouth*

Rubber dam is the most effective technique for isolating teeth, particularly for long-term isolation, during treatment. Introduced in the USA in 1864 it has been extensively used since then by dentists who aim to provide treatment of a high standard.

The principle is that the crowns of one or more teeth project through a sheet of rubber so that the dentist may work on them in isolation from the rest of the mouth.

Advantages of rubber dam   Rubber dam produces effective isolation of one or more teeth from the rest of the oral cavity and thus gives a clean, dry area in which the dentist can work free from saliva, gingival fluid and the intrusion of the tongue and lips. Air breathed by the patient is excluded and visibility is optimal. The dam effectively prevents the ingestion or inhalation of foreign bodies associated with dental treatment, such as fragments of fillings or teeth, castings, crowns or small instruments, particularly those used in endodontic treatment. This is particularly valuable during treatment in the low-seated position when such accidents are likely to happen. The soft tissues are protected from the effects of irritant chemicals such as may be used in endodontic treatment and the bleaching of teeth. The application of rubber dam occupies some time but once it is in position the dentist can proceed with his work more rapidly and with greater security. Most dental restorations are adversely affected to some extent by the presence of moisture; rubber dam, with its effective isolation, avoids this common cause of inferior restorations. It comes nearer than any other method of isolation to providing an environment for the effective control of bacteria which is desirable in endodontic treatment.

Disadvantages of rubber dam   Rubber dam can be applied by an experienced dentist in most cases within a few minutes. In awkward cases the procedure may be more time-consuming. Difficulties arise particularly when teeth are not fully erupted, when they are irregularly placed and when they are tightly in contact over a wide area. The careless application of clamps and ligatures may cause trauma to the gingival tissues. Many patients dislike the use of rubber dam but, if convinced of its value, are prepared to tolerate it. With apprehensive patients it is more important to build up the patient's confidence than to produce a perfect restoration and so the dentist's enthusiasm must be tempered.

Fig. 11.5 Mask type of rubber dam.

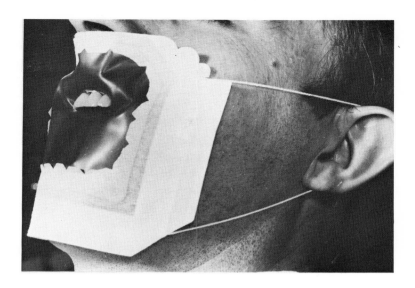

Types of rubber dam

Several types of rubber dam are available commercially.

Mask rubber dam　This consists of a piece of rubber, bordered by a frame of stiff paper to which are attached elastic loops for fixing around the patient's ears (Fig. 11.5). It is of most value in the upper anterior teeth.

Sheet rubber dam　This is marketed in rolls about 15 cm wide and in several grades from light to heavy. It usually requires to be maintained in position by clamps fitting on to the necks of the teeth. The periphery of the rubber is stretched on to the points of the rubber dam frame to permit visibility and access to the teeth (Fig. 11.6). While this is less expensive than the mask type it takes longer to apply and may cause more discomfort.

Equipment used

Rubber dam punch　This is required for punching circular holes in the rubber and gives a range of about six sizes of hole (Fig. 11.7). The smallest size is suitable for a lower incisor and the largest foɪ a first molar. The holes in the punch should be kept sharp so that a circle of rubber is removed cleanly, otherwise the rubber may tear on application.

Fig. 11.6 Sheet rubber dam in position.

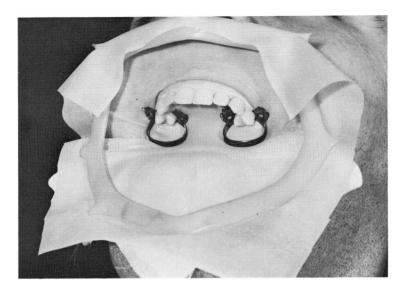

Fig. 11.7 Rubber dam punch with an enlarged view of the head.

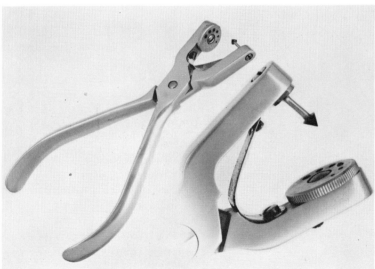

Rubber dam clamps　A range of clamps is available for use when necessary to maintain the rubber in position (Fig. 11.8). Most clamps have two jaws connected by a single bow spring; a few have a double bow. The jaws are concave so as to fit on the buccal and lingual sides of the neck of a tooth. The size and shape of the concavity is related to the tooth for which it is designed. Each jaw has a circular hole into which can be fitted one beak of a pair of

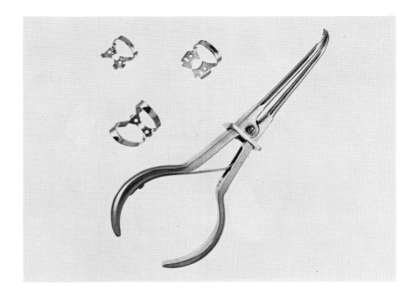

clamp forceps. Usually each jaw has also a small wing. It is wise for the dentist to limit his selection of clamps since a large range is available on the market.

Clamp forceps   The beaks of these are inserted into the holes in the bodies of each clamp; the handles are pressed together to stretch the clamp, and released when it is in position on the tooth. A locking ring enables the clamp to be left on the forceps ready for use. The forceps must be used again for removing the clamp.

Rubber dam frame   A metal or plastic frame is used to stretch the rubber so that the tongue and cheeks are retracted and access to the field of operation is satisfactory (Fig. 11.9).

Technique of using rubber dam

Mask rubber dam   This type of dam is most suited to the anterior teeth and for application to several teeth rather than to a single tooth.

● Holes of a suitable size are punched, using a rubber dam punch, at the points indicated on the paper, and the paper tear-out is removed. Alternatively, the central paper tear-out can be removed and the holes punched freehand (Fig. 11.10).

205   *Control of fluids in the mouth*

Fig. 11.9 Rubber dam frame.

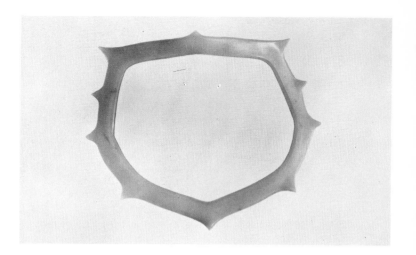

● A piece of dental floss is slipped between the teeth to be included so as to ease the contacts and facilitate the placing of the dam (Fig. 11.11).
● The dam is held with the middle fingers of each hand buccally and lingually to the holes and is slipped on to one tooth at a time, the interdental strips of rubber sliding through the contact areas (Fig. 11.12).
● The elastic ear loops are stretched over the patient's ears.
● The free edges of the rubber at the neck of each tooth to be restored are everted into the gingival sulcus using a plastic-filling instrument. It is often possible to achieve this eversion as the rubber is put in position without the need for subsequent instrumentation.

It is not usually necessary to apply clamps, but if so they should be applied at this stage. Often the rubber will remain in position clear of the gingival margin of a cavity to be restored without assistance, but where it does not, a floss ligature may be applied (Fig. 11.13). A loop is made with a double hitch and this is placed around the tooth, passed through the contact areas on either side, and the hitch is tightened until the waxed floss remains in position below the maximum convexity of the tooth and the gingival margin of the cavity. A plastic-filling instrument may be used to assist this. Finally, the knot is completed.

If the patient finds it more convenient a small suction tube may be inserted under the dam but this is usually of little value when the patient is in the horizontal position.

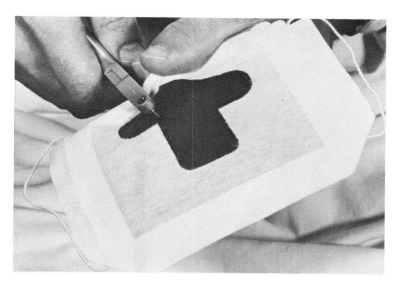

Fig. 11.10 Punching holes in mask
type rubber dam.

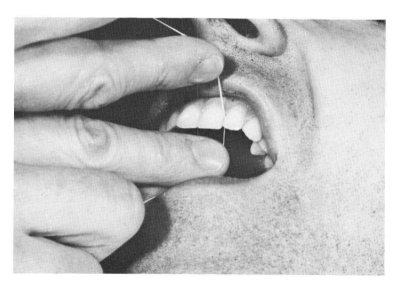

Fig. 11.11 Easing contacts between
teeth with dental floss prior to
application of rubber dam.

207 *Control of fluids in the mouth*

Fig. 11.12 Application of the dam.

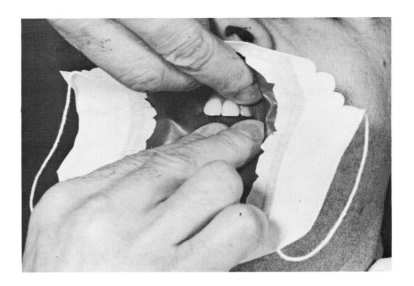

Sheet rubber dam

● A piece of rubber of suitable size is cut from the roll. A 15 cm square is useful for most teeth but for molar teeth a longer piece may be required.

● The sites for punching holes can be located by placing a template on the rubber and marking with a ballpoint pen the position of the teeth to be included. This technique is not satisfactory where the teeth are irregular or where the necks are very close or very far apart. A second method of marking is to position the rubber in the mouth, lightly stretched over the teeth, and place a mark with a ballpoint pen over the centre of each tooth to be included. A skilled operator usually locates the sites on the basis of his experience using neither template nor pen.

● The holes are punched with the rubber dam punch, using a size comparable to the circumference at the neck of the tooth.

● It will be assumed that the teeth are free from plaque and calculus prior to application of the rubber. Where teeth are close together the contacts should be eased by slipping a piece of floss carefully through each one in turn. The rubber is applied by holding it with the middle fingers of each hand buccally and lingually on either side of the holes, pointing towards the teeth and stretching the rubber. Each hole in turn is slipped over the appropriate tooth and the interdental strips of rubber passed through the contacts down to the gingival margin. The rubber is gradually released, if possible leaving the edges of the rubber

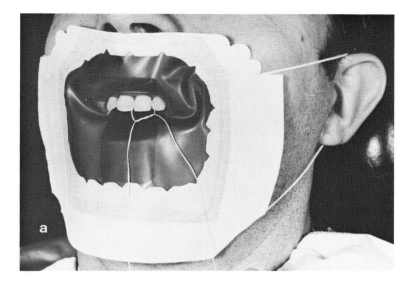

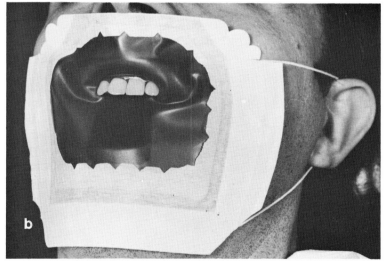

everted into the gingival sulcus. If this is not possible the eversion must be done subsequently with a plastic filling instrument. This is particularly important where the cavity is adjacent to the gingival margin. The number of teeth included depends on the operation to be carried out. For endodontic treatment one tooth should be included; for a single approximal restoration the adjacent tooth should be included and for multiple restorations a group of teeth must be dammed.

209   *Control of fluids in the mouth*

● Sometimes the rubber will remain in a satisfactory position without further aid, but usually it will have to be retained by rubber dam clamps, wooden wedges or ligatures of dental floss. Where clamps are to be used the appropriate clamp is positioned on to the clamp forceps in such a way that the single bow will be towards the posterior part of the mouth. The handles of the forceps are pressed together to stretch the clamp and this is carefully eased over the convexity of the tooth and gently released making sure that it does not close on the gingival tissues but ensuring that it is below the maximum convexity of the tooth in order that it should be retained. When applying the rubber to a group of anterior teeth it is often useful to clamp the premolar teeth since the convexities on their buccal and lingual surfaces facilitate retention of the clamp. It is not essential to fit the clamp directly on to the tooth; this can be done with the rubber intervening.

● Finally, the rubber must be stretched and its periphery fixed on to the points of a rubber dam frame. If necessary, ligatures are placed and, if the patient desires, a small suction tube is put in position. Silicate restorations already present should be coated with a suitable varnish without delay so as to prevent drying and irreversible damage to the material.

Where single teeth, particularly molar teeth, are to be dammed another technique is possible. After perforation the rubber is stretched over the wings of a clamp orientated in the correct position. The clamp forceps are applied to the clamp and this is placed in position on the tooth together with the rubber, and the forceps carefully removed. Finally, the rubber is slipped from each wing of the clamp by means of a plastic-filling instrument until it fits tightly around the neck of the tooth.

Removal of rubber dam

Clamps and ligatures should be removed first. The interdental strips of rubber related to approximal restorations which have just been inserted should be stretched out labially and cut with scissors, being careful not to damage the soft tissues. Finally, the rubber is removed together with the frame and the area irrigated with a water spray.

SYSTEMIC ANTI-SIALAGOGUES

Where the flow of saliva is particularly copious it may occasionally be thought necessary to use a systemic anti-sialagogue drug. Atropine sulphate, given orally $\frac{1}{2}$–1 hour before treatment, is usually effective in reducing salivary secretion. However, the dry sensation in the mouth may be unpleasant for patients and there may be side effects such as blurred vision, so it is preferable to avoid the use of such drugs and to use alternative methods of saliva control.

Chapter 12
Care of the dental pulp
and gingival tissues

Care of the dental pulp

The operator who practises conservative dentistry must be continually aware that the teeth which he treats are vital tissues susceptible to injury. He must consider the condition of the dental pulp and either maintain its healthy state or, if it is diseased, carry out treatment to restore its health and that of the periapical tissues if they have been affected. Unfortunately, even the most accessible part of the dental pulp, in the crown of the tooth, is normally surrounded by a substantial thickness of hard tissue and this leads to considerable difficulty in forming a precise diagnosis of its condition.

As in other parts of the body, the basic principles of inflammation in response to injury apply, but they are modified by special circumstances. The pulp may be considered as an end-organ and is vulnerable to interference with its blood supply. It is surrounded by specialised cells and hard tissue which are not found in other parts of the body, and these modify the basic inflammatory changes which occur. The ground substance of the pulp is highly polymerised and resists the spread of inflammation until it is depolymerised (Bender 1978). Generally, inflammation spreads slowly in the pulp and any increase in pressure is localised. In spite of these features the dental pulp is capable of responding to injury and undergoing repair to a greater extent than was once thought possible, particularly if the apex is still incompletely formed.

In recent years attention has been focussed on the surface of the dentine after cavity preparation. This surface is covered by a layer of smeared dentine and grinding debris. Cavity cleansers have been suggested to remove this layer in order to improve the possible adhesion of some lining and filling materials. Removal of the smear widely opens the entrances to the dentinal tubules. At present the value of cavity cleansers is in question because of the feeling that the open tubules may make the pulp more vulnerable to chemical irritation from materials and to access of micro-organisms (Shortall 1981).

The other area of crucial importance is the margin of the restoration and there is now considerable evidence that micro-organisms may penetrate around and underneath the restoration if the marginal seal is not satisfactory. The presence of these micro-organisms can give rise to inflammation in the pulp as a result of the passage of their toxins along the dentinal tubules. Thus it is desirable to have a liner or base which will adapt closely to the floor of the cavity and prevent the ingress of bacteria, or to have an effective seal at the margin of the restoration, or preferably to have both of these conditions present.

SOURCES OF PULP DAMAGE

Dental caries

This is the most common cause of damage to the dental pulp. There is controversy as to the stage at which dental caries first produces a pulp reaction, but general agreement that irreversible changes in the pulp occur only when caries has approached very close to it.

Impact trauma

Impact injury may produce pulp damage, either through fracture of the tooth exposing the dentine or the pulp itself, or through injury which results in tearing of the apical vessels.

Accidental pulp exposure

Operative procedures resulting in the unplanned exposure of a healthy intact pulp will produce damage, both as a result of the introduction of micro-organisms and through direct trauma to the pulp tissues.

Thermal trauma

This may occur through high-speed preparation of teeth without adequate cooling, which produces a rise in temperature in the dentine (Shovelton & Marsland 1960; Langeland 1961; Morrant & Kramer 1963). Thermal trauma may occur through metal fillings placed deeply into the dentine without adequate insulation.

Chemical and bacterial trauma

Some filling materials and cements cause pulpal inflammation and at one time this was believed to be due to chemical action. More recently there has been evidence that bacterial irritation may be the main cause (Brännström & Nyborg 1971). Bacteria can be demonstrated in spaces between the restoration and the walls and floor of the cavity and even in the dentinal tubules, but there is not a high correlation between their presence and pulp inflammation (Skogedal & Eriksen 1976).

Desiccation

Drying of dentine through prolonged use of an air jet may produce pulp damage (Brännström 1968).

HISTOPATHOLOGICAL CHANGES IN THE PULP

Some sources of pulp damage, such as cavity preparation, occur relatively rapidly and so tend to present a characteristic pattern representing early changes in response to injury. Other sources of damage, such as caries, act relatively slowly over a longer period and hence show mainly chronic changes.

Early changes in the pulp in response to injury include:

● The passage of odontoblast nuclei into the dentinal tubules (Fig. 12.1).
● Oedema, disruption and cellular infiltration of the odontoblast layer (Fig. 12.2).
● Infiltration of inflammatory cells deep into the pulp (Fig. 12.3).
● Haemorrhage into the pulp.

These changes are found primarily opposite tubules leading from the area of the injury. The nature and severity of the changes may be influenced by factors such as the thickness and the nature of the dentine overlying the pulp and the period of time which has elapsed since the trauma.

Late changes in the dental pulp depend on the success of the defence mechanisms. If these are able to cope with the injury the early changes will be reversed, the inflammation will resolve, the haemorrhage will be replaced by fibrous tissue and reparative changes will take place in the dentine. These changes include the formation of reparative secondary dentine along the pulpal border of the primary dentine and the formation of peritubular dentine

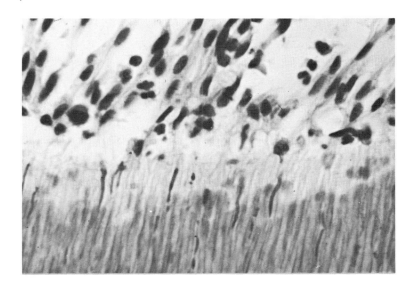

Fig. 12.1 Odontoblast nuclei in the dentinal tubules 2 days after insertion of a silicate filling without a lining.

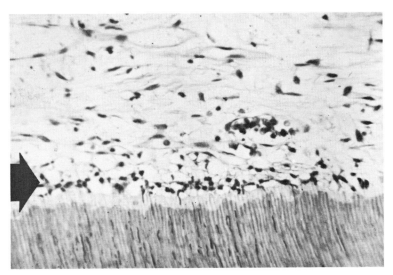

Fig. 12.2 Disrupted odontoblast layer (*arrow*) 7 days after preparation of a cavity using an air turbine without cooling.

resulting in a narrowing or occlusion of the tubules to form an area of sclerosed dentine. In any event, odontoblast nuclei disappear from the tubules within a period of several weeks as the result of autolysis.

If, however, the injury is too severe for the defence mechanisms to cope with, or is progressive as in the case of untreated caries, degenerative changes will take place.

215 *Care of the dental pulp and gingival tissues*

Fig. 12.3 Inflammatory cell infiltration deep in the coronal pulp 98 days after insertion of a silicate filling without a lining.

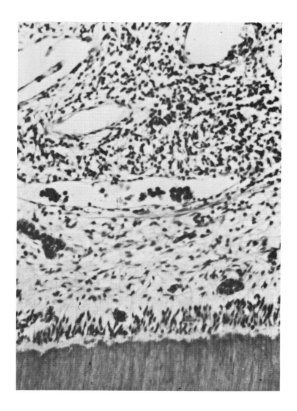

DIAGNOSIS OF PULP DISEASE

Such diagnosis of pulp condition as can be made should be based on information obtained from a careful history and examination.

History

Full details of the history relating to the tooth in question should be obtained as set out in Chapter 3.

Clinical examination

The colour of the tooth may be an important diagnostic feature. A darkening of the crown may indicate death of the pulp; a yellowish discoloration suggests calcification of the coronal part of the pulp. The presence and superficial extent of caries and restorations should be assessed, noting whether the restorations are satisfactory particularly around their margins. Tenderness on percussion may indicate an inflammatory reaction of the apical pulp or the periapical region or the presence of a periapical abscess. Mobility may indicate periodontitis originating from a damaged pulp but this must be differentiated from the effects of periodontal disease and traumatic periodontitis.

Transillumination

Transillumination of teeth is carried out by viewing the labial surface of the tooth in darkened surroundings having placed a small light on the lingual surface. If transillumination shows a pink colour the pulp may be vital; if it looks dark pulp death may have occurred.

Radiography

Bitewing radiographs are essential to show clearly the crowns of the upper and lower posterior teeth and periapical views are required to show the condition of the periapical hard tissues. Radiographs may give some indication of the depth of caries, the presence of caries undiagnosed at clinical examination, caries under a restoration, the absence of a lining under a radiolucent restoration, extensive reparative secondary dentine or, in the case of periapical radiographs, a periapical radiolucency which may originate from a necrotic pulp. Changes in the soft tissues of the pulp do not, of course, show on a radiograph.

Pulp testing

Pulp testing is perhaps an unfortunate term since it implies a greater degree of success than is usually obtained. Nevertheless, the response of the pulp to electrical, hot and cold stimuli may provide valuable information concerning pulp vitality.

Electric pulp testing is carried out using an electric pulp tester. This apparatus provides a means of applying an electric current to the surface of the crown of a tooth and, by conduction through the enamel and the dentine, stimulating the pulp and producing a pain response. The object is to obtain information about the vitality of the pulp.

The tooth is isolated and dried carefully to avoid conduction through a film of saliva on the crown which might stimulate the pain receptors in the gingival and periodontal tissues and give a false response. In one type (Fig. 12.4) the patient holds the hand electrode while the tooth electrode, bearing a small quantity of

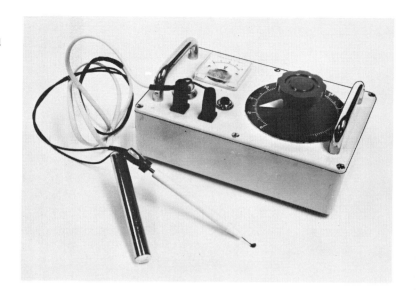

Fig. 12.4 Electric pulp tester. The circular dial is part of a rheostat which controls the voltage. The metal cylinder is held in the patient's hand and the wire loop at the end of an insulating handle is applied to the tooth.

electrode jelly or similar substance to improve electrical contact, is applied to the labial or buccal surface remote from the gingiva and from any fillings, particularly metal fillings. The voltage, previously set at zero, is slowly increased until pain is experienced by the patient or the maximum current is reached without pain. In the former case the threshold reading at which pain first occurs, is noted; in the latter case a negative response is recorded. When pain occurs the electrode is removed promptly. Neither the operator's fingers nor the patient's soft tissues should contact the uninsulated part of the active electrode.

The effect of thermal stimuli on the tooth can be determined by applying a pledget of cotton wool, which has been sprayed with ethyl chloride, on to the crown of the tooth. If a pain response is obtained the stimulus is removed at once. In a similar way a stick of gutta percha may be heated at one end and applied to the crown of the tooth to test pulp reaction to hot stimuli. The significance of a positive reaction to electrical or thermal stimuli will be discussed later but for the present it is sufficient to point out that the thermal stimuli applied as described are crude and cannot be quantified. Perhaps the most effective indication of pulp vitality is the occurrence of pain on cutting dentine. Where pulp vitality is in doubt and some preparation of the tooth is required it may be best to commence this without local anaesthesia in the hope of confirming a previous diagnosis regarding pulp vitality.

There are at present many classifications of pulp disease based on histopathology, and a real need exists for standardisation. The classification to be described follows that of Seltzer & Bender (1975).

Atrophic pulp

This pulp condition shows much fibrous tissue with a reduction in the number of cells and extensive secondary dentine.

Acute pulpitis

This usually occurs as a sequel to operative procedures and gives a picture of odontoblast changes, blood vessels dilated, haemorrhages and the presence of acute inflammatory cells. The condition is usually localised and of short duration since it either heals or progresses to chronic inflammation. This term is used in a histological sense and does not imply the existence of acute pain. In fact, pain is uncommon in this condition.

Transitional pulpitis

In this condition, chronic inflammatory cells are present but not in sufficient quantity to be regarded as a chronic pulpitis. It is likely to be found under deep caries and sometimes after traumatic operative procedures.

Chronic partial pulpitis

This condition may develop under deep caries, pulp exposures and traumatic operative procedures. Part of the pulp is extensively infiltrated with chronic inflammatory cells, particularly plasma cells and lymphocytes. This lesion may be walled off by fibrous tissue and the remaining pulp may be relatively normal.

Chronic partial pulpitis with partial necrosis

Not infrequently a small region of liquefaction necrosis develops within an area of chronic inflammation in the pulp.

Chronic total pulpitis

The entire pulp is inflamed and frequently the inflammation has spread to the periodontal tissues at the apex. An area of pulp necrosis exists.

Total necrosis

The pulp is completely necrotic and the periapical tissues show evidence of inflammation.

Clearly this classification is an over-simplification since many variations exist but it may have value in helping the student to understand the progressive nature of the processes of pulp pathology.

Accurate diagnosis of pulp condition is very difficult without extraction of the tooth and in a multi-rooted tooth the pulp condition may be different in the several roots. It is equally true that, even if a pulp condition could be diagnosed, we still do not have sufficient knowledge to assess the prognosis accurately. Nevertheless, the clinician must attempt to make not a histological but a clinical diagnosis. His assessment will be most accurate if it is based on knowledge of the correlations between clinical findings and pathological states. In particular he will need to assess to which one of three groups a pulp belongs at any time:

A A pulp which will remain healthy or return to health if the irritant is removed and a non-irritant dressing placed.

B A pulp which will not return to a healthy state even after removal of the irritant and insertion of a dressing.

C A pulp which may return to health following treatment but about which the prognosis is uncertain.

In the first group it will be possible to maintain the vitality and restore the health of the pulp. In the second group, part or all of the pulp will need to be removed or the tooth extracted in order to restore the health of the tissues. In the third group the irritant should be removed, a dressing inserted and a final diagnosis delayed until a future occasion when allocation to the first or second group is possible.

CORRELATION BETWEEN CLINICAL FINDINGS AND HISTOPATHOLOGY

Possible correlations of this type have been investigated by several workers, notably by Seltzer & Bender (1975), but the correlation values are rarely high and this contributes to the difficulty of diagnosis.

Pain

In teeth with extensive caries the presence of pain is highly correlated with the presence of a pulp exposure. Severe pain is most likely to occur in partial pulpitis with partial necrosis. Unfortunately, the character of the pain does not appear to be of much diagnostic value. The severity is important and as a generalisation it can be said that, where there has been severe pain for as long as one day, the changes are probably irreversible. The occurrence of pain on thermal or other stimuli appears to be of little diagnostic value.

Pain on percussion

Pain on percussion is more frequently found in cases where necrosis, either partial or total, is present and so percussion is a test with some diagnostic value.

Electric and thermal testing

The electric pulp test which produces no response is of considerable value in indicating the probability of complete necrosis of the pulp, provided that it has been carried out under carefully controlled conditions. Threshold values are of much less significance in diagnosing phases of pulp disease (Mumford 1967). The crude nature of testing with gutta percha and ethyl chloride means they are of little value as diagnostic procedures. The literature is reviewed by Chambers (1982).

Radiographic examination

The correlation between the presence of a periapical radiolucency and the histological demonstration of a periapical granuloma is only moderately high. There is also some degree of examiner variability in the identification of periapical pathology (Goldman, Pearson & Darzenta 1972). Both these factors mean that, while radiographic examination is valuable, it is by no means an infallible diagnostic measure.

TREATMENT OF A TRAUMATIC EXPOSURE OF A
HEALTHY PULP

The pulp may be unintentionally exposed during preparation of a tooth and in some cases it may be advisable to undertake pulp capping. This involves isolating the tooth, preferably with rubber dam, and placing a dressing on the pulp, usually of calcium hydroxide. A base or temporary dressing is subsequently placed on it. The success of this procedure is higher if the exposure is not infected by saliva or caries, but in any event careful follow-up is indicated.

TREATMENT OF DEEP CARIES IN A TOOTH WITH A
HEALTHY PULP

It should be clear from the preceding pages that the treatment of pulp disease depends to a large extent on a correct assessment of its condition. One of the most common clinical decisions which has to be made in conservative dentistry is the decision as to whether deep caries should be completely removed or not. It can be stated as an inviolable rule that all shallow caries ought to be removed. At one time it was widely held, particularly in the USA, that all deep caries should also be removed even though this might result in a pulp exposure. It was also standard practice to treat the cavity with antiseptics in order to ensure that no micro-organisms would remain on the floor and that no further progress of caries would occur. Others denied the need to remove all soft dentine and believed that if it were 'sealed in' by a filling, caries would not advance (Kraus 1945).

It is now current practice, supported by some research work (Jordan & Suzuki 1971), to leave a small amount of deep carious dentine if its removal is thought likely to produce an exposure of the pulp, provided that—and this is most important—the pulp is deemed likely to return to good health (Group A). This technique is known as *indirect pulp capping*. It should be clearly understood that no shallow caries may be left or more than a small amount of slightly soft deep dentine. The deep part of the cavity should then be covered by calcium hydroxide or zinc oxide–eugenol, and the tooth restored either immediately or on a subsequent visit. Calcium hydroxide is to be preferred because of its property of stimulating dentine sclerosis and secondary dentine formation (Geller, Klein & McDonald 1971). It is wise to explain to the patient or parent that the tooth is on probation and that, should symptoms occur, the dentist should be consulted.

Some authors advise that such cavities should be temporarily restored and re-opened after a period of several months for the removal of all soft caries but it has yet to be demonstrated that this second stage is necessary. On account of the variability in the rate of secondary dentine formation (Corbett 1963) there would seem to be some risk of exposing a viable pulp at this stage.

Guidelines for the use of indirect pulp capping technique

● All shallow caries must be removed.
● All very soft, deep caries must be removed.
● The pulp must be judged as either healthy or capable of a return to health.
● There must be no actual exposure present.
● The patient should be advised to report if symptoms occur.
● Radiographic follow-up after 1 year is desirable.

TREATMENT OF A DISEASED PULP IN A TOOTH WITH
DEEP CARIES

The first stage is to use the information obtained from the history and examination to assess the pulp condition as far as is possible. The student should understand that it is possible to give only general guidelines owing to the difficulty of making an accurate diagnosis. An attempt must be made to allocate the pulp to Groups A, B or C as described above.

Group A, in which the pulp is able to return to health, includes atrophic pulpitis, acute pulpitis, transitional pulpitis and the early stages of chronic partial pulpitis. These cases will generally have given rise to little or no pain and not to severe pain (Seltzer & Bender 1975). The student should appreciate that acute pulpitis is by no means synonymous with acute pain. In these cases the pulp should be treated by the technique of indirect pulp capping using calcium hydroxide.

Group B, in which the pulp is irreparably damaged, includes chronic partial pulpitis with partial necrosis, chronic total pulpitis and total necrosis. Teeth in this group will generally have given rise to one or more of the following signs and symptoms:

● Severe pain lasting more than one day.
● A negative result to electric pulp testing and to test drilling.
● An apical radiolucency.
● Definite tenderness on percussion which is judged to be of pulpal origin.

If several of these signs and symptoms are present greater confidence can be given to the diagnosis than if only one is present. Teeth in this group may be treated by endodontic therapy and root filling, or by extraction.

Group C includes the early stages of chronic partial pulpitis without the presence of necrosis. Such teeth may have given rise to intermittent pain or severe pain for a few hours at the most. The best results are obtained by excavation of caries leaving only deep caries, provided that it is not very soft. A dressing of calcium hydroxide is inserted and the tooth is kept under observation for a period and in the absence of unfavourable signs or symptoms is restored. If excavation of caries reveals an exposure of the pulp, the tooth should be allocated to Group B and treated by endodontic therapy, extraction or pulpotomy. A pulpal exposure is diagnosed by isolation of the cavity, drying and examination in good light. The point of a probe should be drawn lightly across the floor of the cavity in the region of the pulp horns. If it catches in a hole in the floor a pulp exposure may be diagnosed. There may or may not be haemorrhage. The student should not attempt to push the probe into the floor which might create an exposure nor should he diagnose an exposure unless it is at least 3 mm from the enamel–dentine junction.

Pulpotomy is the surgical removal under aseptic conditions of a portion of the pulp, generally the whole of the coronal pulp, and dressing the surface of the remaining pulp with calcium hydroxide which is then sealed in. The object is to remove all diseased and infected pulp tissue and maintain the vitality and health of the remaining pulp. This technique is therefore indicated where only the surface of the pulp is infected or diseased and the remainder is healthy. Further details of pulp capping and pulpotomy should be sought in a textbook of endodontics.

EFFECTS OF CAVITY PREPARATION

Cavity preparation at very low speeds of the order or 250 r.p.m. produces no changes in the dental pulp. When speeds of 3000–5000 r.p.m. are used without cooling, slight changes may be produced. However, with speeds over 5000 r.p.m. changes indicative of pulp damage are more frequently found. These include aspiration of odontoblast nuclei, oedema and disruption of the odontoblast layer, infiltration of the pulp with inflammatory cells and sometimes haemorrhages. These changes become more marked with increase in speed and areas of pulp necrosis may result. They are due to heat production during cutting and can be avoided or considerably reduced if an effective water spray is used with speeds above 5000 r.p.m.; below this speed water cooling is unnecessary. If excessive pressure is applied when cutting with the air turbine, the bur may stall and cause additional heat production, so this should be avoided (Morrant 1977).

The effects of these materials are usually tested by placing them in Class V cavities, prepared in human premolar teeth scheduled for extraction for orthodontic reasons. The cavities are cut with every precaution to avoid pulp damage and, after filling with the test material, are extracted at set intervals. The pulps are examined histologically.

At one time pulp reaction to materials placed on the dentine of cavity floors was considered to be largely due to chemical irritation and linings were placed under irritant materials with the aim of isolating the dentine surface from them. More recently it has been suspected that micro-organisms on cavity floors may be the major source of irritation. The organisms may be present after cavity preparation, as a result of caries or contamination from the mouth, or they may gain ingress through the poorly fitting margins of a restoration. Linings are still placed under materials which cause pulp irritation but more with a view to excluding or controlling bacterial contamination. It follows that the lining materials should be carefully placed so that they are well adapted to the dentine of the cavity floor. In addition, some authorities recommend the use of cavity cleansers whose purpose is to remove the layer of debris and bacteria which are left on the cavity floor after preparation has been completed.

For many years silicate cement was considered to be one of the most irritant of filling materials and this was attributed to its low pH when inserted. Although seldom used now in clinical practice it has provided the basis for much research into this subject. For example, when the superficial part of a silicate filling was removed soon after its insertion and replaced by zinc oxide and eugenol cement, the pupal response was greatly reduced (Skogedal & Eriksen 1976). They also found a higher frequency of bacteria under silicate fillings in teeth with unacceptable pulp responses, but this was not the case with composite fillings. Bergvall & Brännström (1971) found spaces of from 2 to 20 μm under composite fillings, and about half that width around the walls. Brännström, Vojinovic & Nordenvall (1979) found bacteria growing in the contraction gap between the silicate cement and the cavity walls in a large majority of restorations examined. They concluded that silicate cement *per se* does not seriously irritate the pulp and that it is important to remove grinding debris with an anti-bacterial cavity cleanser and to use a liner to prevent the entrance of bacteria from the mouth.

Liners such as calcium hydroxide are associated with a low

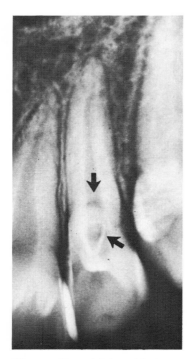

Fig. 12.5 Upper left lateral incisor affected by dens invaginatus. This developmental anomaly arises from the cingulum region and forms an ovoid cavity (*arrows*) lined by dentine and in parts by enamel.

degree of pulpal irritation and there is some evidence that they inhibit the growth and penetration of bacteria (Qvist, Qvist & Lambjerg-Hansen 1977). Under zinc oxide and eugenol there is slight irritation. Of the cementing media, EBA cements and zinc polycarboxylate cements are associated with mild pulpal irritation. Zinc phosphate cement is generally considered to be highly irritant but some disagree with this (Brännström & Nyborg 1977). Temporary crown and bridge materials, such as epimine and self-polymerising acrylic resin, show moderate to severe pulp irritation if placed in cavities without a lining, but are probably less harmful when used with a non-irritant temporary cement. Amalgams, including high copper amalgams, show a slight to moderate pulp response when inserted without a lining and this is followed by the deposition of tubular reparative dentine. Occasionally, particles of tin and zinc may pass into the dentinal tubules. Under composite cements there is a mild to moderate degree of pulp irritation and it is generally recommended that a liner should be placed beneath them.

DENS INVAGINATUS

This is a developmental defect which affects the palatal surfaces of upper lateral incisors and, less frequently, upper central incisors. Clinically, it appears as a pit in the cingulum region which is usually stained and into which a probe may pass so that it resembles a carious cavity. Radiographic examination shows that it is a flask-shape invagination of enamel and dentine into the pulp (Fig. 12.5). It originates as an invagination of the enamel organ prior to the commencement of calcification.

Dens invaginatus is important because of its clinical significance. In the first place, if the condition is not recognised and cavity preparation is commenced, the entrance to the invagination may closely resemble a pulp exposure and the clinician may decide that endodontic treatment is required. However, if the pulp is healthy it need not be disturbed. Instead the lesion may be treated by exposing the invagination, cleaning out the contents and filling it with a suitable non-irritant lining prior to restoration of the cavity.

The second feature of clinical importance is that the enamel and dentine lining the invagination may be deficient so that it connects directly with the pulp. In this event micro-organisms may penetrate to the pulp soon after the tooth erupts into the oral cavity and pulp infection and necrosis may result. Consequently, it is important to make a radiographic examination of the apical region of the tooth prior to its restoration.

Care of the gingival tissues

In the same way that the pulp may be damaged by conservative procedures so the gingival tissues may be affected, either temporarily or permanently. In fact, where restorations contact the gingival tissues, some degree of permanent damage is inevitable. Nevertheless, awareness and care on the part of the dentist may reduce this to a minimum. Removal of plaque and the establishment of effective oral hygiene are essential preparations for any course of conservation treatment. If we were able to effectively prevent dental caries and obviate the need for restorations there is no doubt that a considerable amount of gingival disease would be prevented.

SOURCES OF DAMAGE TO THE GINGIVAL TISSUES

Dental caries

Carious lesions which extend to the gingival margin or sub-gingivally cause gingival irritation and inflammation principally through the action of dental plaque which is impossible to remove.

Operative procedures

The gingivae may be damaged by procedures such as the use of burs and hand instruments, and the careless use of matrix bands and retraction fibre.

Restorations

Restorations and temporary or permanent crowns, which extend to the gingival margin or sub-gingivally, lead to a chronic marginal gingivitis and in fact form one of the primary causes of this condition. Cement, forced sub-gingivally during the insertion of crowns or inlays and not carefully removed, has the same result. This damage is due mainly to dental plaque which is retained by the restorations and is difficult to remove. The gingival irritation is increased if the surface of the restoration is rough or if there is a marginal defect or excess. It becomes more severe the further the restoration extends beneath the free gingival margin (Waerhaug 1960). In these cases the removal of plaque by the patient is not only difficult but impossible. As Löe (1968) has stated: 'From a periodontal viewpoint all margins of gold, porcelain and acrylic crowns may be considered ill-fitting'.

Inadequate contacts

Inadequate contact areas also lead to gingival disease as a result of food impaction and the retention of the fibrous elements of food, and more particularly dental plaque (Gould & Picton 1966).

Chemical effects of restorations

It is possible that some restorative materials are chemically more irritant than others but this is difficult to confirm experimentally. Löe (1968) concluded as a result of surveying the literature that gold, porcelain and heat-cured acrylic were well tolerated by the tissues. Amalgam, silicate and zinc phosphate cement on the other hand were irritant, possibly because of their chemical nature. The significance of phosphate cement is that, when used as a cementing medium for inlays or crowns, it is present to a greater or lesser extent at the margins of these restorations.

RESULTS OF DAMAGE

The various forms of trauma described above lead to inflammation of the gingival tissues. Short-term trauma, such as may be caused by instrumentation will, in the absence of bacterial plaque or further trauma, usually lead to resolution and healing (Löe 1968). However, long-term trauma, produced for example by sub-gingival restorations, may lead to a localised chronic marginal gingivitis (Silness 1970; Mannerberg 1971). This may progress to chronic marginal periodontitis and there is evidence of increased bone loss in the region of restorations with gingival excess (Alexander 1968; Gilmore & Sheiham 1971).

Histopathology

The histological appearance associated with sub-gingival restorations (Fig. 12.6) is typically one of chronic inflammatory cells in the connective tissues beneath the sulcular epithelium. The epithelium is disorganised, thin or absent in some places and shows evidence of hyperplasia in other parts. There may be resorption of the alveolar crest with the associated loss of periodontal fibres.

Fig. 12.6 Gingival tissue adjacent to an amalgam filling (*large space*) in a dog 200 days after insertion of the filling. Note the dense cellular infiltration and the traces of plaque on the cavity flow.

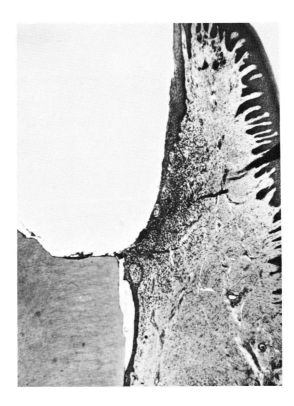

PREVENTION OF DAMAGE TO THE GINGIVAL TISSUES

Removal of dental plaque and calculus and the establishment of good oral hygiene should precede the making of any permanent restorations. This treatment should reduce gingival inflammation to a minimum and allow ulceration of the gingival epithelium to heal, otherwise the effects of any trauma to the gingival tissues will be exacerbated and the resultant haemorrhage may make conservation treatment more difficult. Periodontal and conservation treatment should be co-ordinated so that each is carried out at the best time. In general it is more satisfactory to make permanent restorations after the periodontal treatment has been completed and the gingival tissues rendered healthy. This avoids inconvenience from haemorrhage, gives better access for preparation and, where aesthetics are important, allows the new level of the gingival tissues to become established. On the other hand, the presence of defective contact areas or of gingival excess on restorations may delay healing after gingival surgery and should be corrected in advance.

Burs and hand instruments should be used with considerable care in the region of the gingival tissues to avoid damage or cause only the minimum trauma necessary to obtain a good restoration. Damage by hand cutting instruments may be avoided by the prior retraction of the gingival margin by means of retraction fibre. This method is less satisfactory where rotary instruments are used since the fibre may be entrapped by the bur. Baker-Curson burs are particularly valuable for finishing enamel margins and cause very little gingival damage.

However, with trauma from instrumentation, if local environmental conditions are favourable, healing should take place satisfactorily. It is probably better to accept some degree of short-term trauma of this nature and produce a well-finished restoration than to risk the long-term effects of a poorly finished restoration. The careless use of retraction fibre prior to taking an impression may cause tearing of the gingival attachment and result in permanent and unsightly recession. The fibre used should not be too thick and should not be pressed out of sight into the sulcus. Astringent chemicals are harmful and should rarely be used.

Preparations should not be extended sub-gingivally except for the removal of caries or for aesthetic reasons. It was the teaching of Black (1908) and his successors that the gingival margins of cavities should be extended sub-gingivally in order to avoid the risk of future caries in this region. However, now that we are aware of the damage to the gingival tissues which can result from this policy, opinion has changed and it is now believed that cavities should not be extended sub-gingivally for prevention but only where caries is actually present (Orban & Mueller 1929; Waerhaug 1960; Löe 1968). However, this policy does carry with it the need to ensure that patients practise effective hygiene, particularly interdental hygiene, by irrigation, dental floss or wood points.

Restorations in the region of the gingival tissues should be smooth and well polished and have well-adapted margins free from gingival excess so as to give optimum opportunity for removal of plaque by patients. Restorations should have the correct contour on the buccal and lingual surfaces and firm approximal contacts of the correct contour should be established. Poorly contoured approximal areas may allow food impaction, particularly where there is an opposing cusp, and this may lead to marginal gingivitis and pocketing. Over-contouring of buccal and lingual surfaces may lead to difficulty in cleansing; under-contouring is probably less harmful. After any approximal restoration is completed the surface should be swept with floss to ensure that cleaning by the patient is practicable.

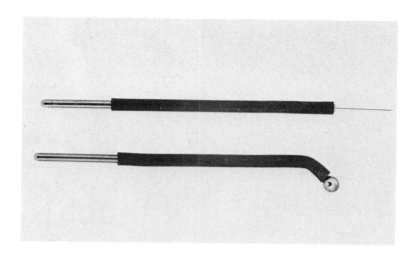

Control of gingival haemorrhage

In spite of all the measures suggested above, gingival haemorrhage will still occur on occasions, such as after the removal of a restoration with gingival excess or where a cavity extends some distance sub-gingivally. In such cases, control of haemorrhage should be instituted before proceeding with cavity preparation, otherwise work will be difficult. In any event, this will have to be controlled before the filling is inserted. Pressure on the bleeding area with a cotton wool pledget soaked in a 1:1000 aqueous solution of adrenalin, or injection of a local anaesthetic containing adrenalin into the base of the gingival papilla may successfully avert further haemorrhage, but electrosurgery is the method of choice for all but minor bleeding.

Electrosurgery involves the passage of high-frequency electrical current through the tissues resulting in a localised heating of the area. Two modes are used in the control of gingival haemorrhage, electrosection for cutting away excess soft tissue, and electrocoagulation for stopping surface bleeding. The area should be anaesthetised and isolated. An indifferent electrode plate is beneath the patient's shoulder, outside the clothing so long as this is not thick. A thin wire electrode is used as the active electrode for cutting and a heavy rounded electrode for coagulation (Fig. 12.7). The correct setting should be chosen on the machine (Fig. 12.8). For cutting, the wire electrode is stroked evenly, without stopping and without pressure, across the base of the area to be cut. This is repeated as necessary, cleaning the electrode between strokes until

231   *Care of the dental pulp and gingival tissues*

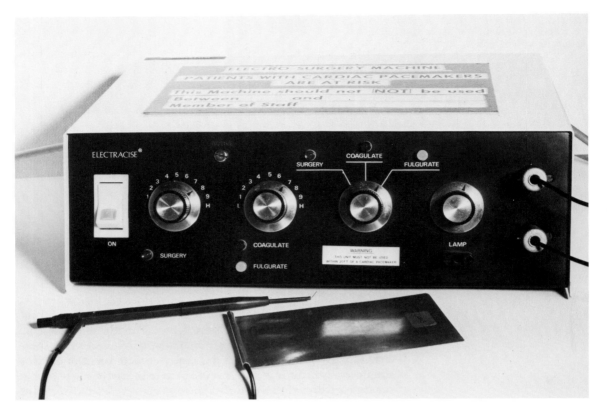

Fig. 12.8 Electrosurgery machine
with active electrode in handle and
indifferent electrode plate.

the excess tissue is separated off. Pausing in the middle of a stroke
will cause the heat to spread into healthy tissue; failure to clean the
electrode will inhibit the passage of the current.

In coagulation the heavy electrode is pressed against the
surface, after this has been swabbed dry, for 2–3 seconds only, and
the effects observed. This may need to be repeated but prolonged
contact is dangerous as the coagulation will damage deeper tissue.
An unpleasant smell results from electrosurgery and it is kind to
remove this with suction. Used with consideration it need not be
unpleasant for the patient and with skill it effectively clears the
area and controls haemorrhage prior to conservation treatment. It
should never be used near a patient who has had a cardiac
pacemaker fitted.

Astringent chemicals, such as zinc and aluminium chlorides,
were formerly applied topically to control gingival haemorrhage
but have been superseded by electrosurgery.

Dentine hypersensitivity

Patients sometimes complain of hypersensitivity or pain induced by thermal changes or sweet foods which is associated with an exposed area of dentine at the neck of the tooth. The area becomes exposed following recession of the gingivae and abrasion of the thin layer of cement overlying the dentine of the root. These areas occur most frequently on the buccal surfaces of the teeth, have a polished appearance and are often associated with the effects of abrasion in patients who use a heavy horizontal brushing action. The condition may also arise as the result of erosion, or following a gingivectomy in which extensive areas of the root may become exposed.

The diagnosis is usually simple since the patient can localise the source, and the careful application of a gentle stream of air will usually reveal the sensitive area. The student should avoid direct probing of these areas with instruments since this can be most painful. According to the hydrodynamic theory sensation in dentine is associated with a movement of fluid in the tubules. In dentine which has been exposed in the mouth for some time and which is not subject to abrasion or acid, the superficial ends of the dentinal tubules become blocked and are not a source of discomfort. However, with continued abrasion or erosion the tubules remain open and the patient finds the area sensitive.

Most of the attempts to reduce sensitivity have been directed at blocking the entrances to the tubules. Astringent chemicals, such as 10 per cent zinc chloride, have been used and produce a very limited improvement in some cases. Rather more effective is the topical application of a siloxane ester which, it is claimed, is capable of impregnating the surface layer of the dentine without producing pulp damage. The technique of application is to isolate and dry the teeth as painlessly as possible and apply the liquid to the sensitive area using a pledget of cotton wool. The surface is kept moistened with the liquid for several minutes. Several applications of the agent may be required. Recently, Brännström, Vojinovic & Nordenvall (1979) have attempted to block the entrances to the tubules by flowing in a quick-setting resin material but the presence of dentinal fluid makes this difficult. Another approach is the use of desensitising dentifrices containing strontium chloride or formalin. These can be used like a normal toothpaste or applied to the sensitive areas on the tip of a finger. In any case, the correction of faulty brushing technique and avoidance of acid foods and drinks is a wise precaution.

References and further reading

ALEXANDER A.G. (1968) *Brit. dent. J.* **125**, 111–114.

BENDER I.B. (1978) *J. Endodont.* **4**, 37–52.

BERGVALL O. & BRÄNNSTRÖM M. (1971) *Swed. dent. J.* **64**, 217–226.

BLACK G.V. (1908) *Operative Dentistry. Pathology of the Hard Tissues of the Teeth*, Vol. 1. Medico-Dental Publishing Co., Chicago.

BRÄNNSTRÖM M. (1968) *J. pros. Dent.* **20**, 165–171.

BRÄNNSTRÖM M. & NORDENVALL K.J. (1978) *J. dent. Res.* **57** (1), 3–10.

BRÄNNSTRÖM M. & NYBORG H. (1971) *Swed. dent. J.* **64**, 149–155.

BRÄNNSTRÖM M. & NYBORG H. (1977) *J. Amer. dent. Ass.* **94**, 308–310.

BRÄNNSTRÖM M., VOJINOVIC O. & NORDENVALL K.J. (1979) *J. Prosthet. dent.* **41**, 290–294.

CHAMBERS I.G. (1982) *Internl. endodont. J.* **15**, 1–5.

CORBETT M.E. (1963) *Brit. dent. J.* **114**, 142–147.

FRANK R.M. (1975) *J. dent. Res.* **54** (B), 176–187.

GELLER J.S., KLEIN A.I. & McDONALD R.E. (1971) *J. Amer. dent. Ass.* **83**, 118–124.

GILMORE N. & SHEIHAM A. (1971) *J. Periodont.* **42**, 8–12.

GOLDMAN M., PEARSON A.H. & DARZENTA N. (1972) *Oral Surg.* **33**, 432–437.

GOULD M.S.E. & PICTON D.C.A. (1966) *Brit. dent. J.* **121**, 20–23.

JORDAN R.E. & SUZUKI M. (1971) *J. Canad. dent. Ass.* **37**, 337–342.

KRAUS A. (1945) *Brit. dent. J.* **78**, 230–237.

LANGELAND K. (1961) *Oral Surg.* **14**, 210–233.

LÖE H. (1968) *Int. dent. J.* **18**, 759–778.

MANNERBERG F. (1971) *Odont. Rev.* **22**, 155–162.

MORRANT G.A. (1977) *J. Br. Endodont. Soc.* **10**, 3–8.

MORRANT G.A. & KRAMER I. (1963) *Brit. dent. J.* **115**, 99–110.

MUMFORD J.M. (1967) *Proc. Roy. Soc. Med.* **60**, 197–200.

ORBAN B. & MUELLER E. (1929) *J. Amer. dent. Ass.* **16**, 1206–1242.

QVIST J., QVIST V. & LAMBJERG-HANSEN H. (1977) *Scand. J. dent. Res.* **85**, 313–319.

SELTZER S. & BENDER I.B. (1975) *The Dental Pulp: Biologic Considerations in Dental Procedures.* 2nd ed. Lippincott, Philadelphia.

SHORTALL A. (1981) *Brit. dent. J.* **150**, 243–247.

SHOVELTON D.S. & MARSLAND E.A. (1960) *Brit. dent. F.* **109**, 225–234.

SILNESS J. (1970) *J. Periodont. Res.* **5**, 219–229.

SKOGEDAL O. & ERIKSEN H.M. (1976) *Scand. J. dent. Res.* **84**, 381–385.

WAERHAUG J. (1960) *Dent. Clin. N. Amer.* March, 161–176.

Chapter 13
Sterilisation and hygiene

An important part of the dentist's responsibility to his patients is to provide dental care in safe, pleasant and hygienic surroundings. This implies that the premises and equipment should be clean and tidy and that the dental personnel should impress patients by their neatness and high standards of personal hygiene. Every effort should be made to prevent cross-infection.

CROSS-INFECTION

Cross-infection may take place from one patient to another, from dentist to patient or from patient to dentist. Surgery assistant and technicians may, less frequently, transmit or receive infection. Cross-infection from one patient to another may occur through the medium of instruments, the hands of the dentist or through contact of the dentist's hands with previously contaminated equipment. Droplet infection may occur through coughing and sneezing. Spray from the air turbine or triple syringe may carry micro-organisms from the patient's mouth into the atmosphere but efficient use of the aspirator will reduce this risk. Polishing of the teeth may also spread droplets containing micro-organisms.

It is difficult to evaluate the frequency with which cross-infection occurs in dental practice or indeed its results. If pathogenic organisms are transferred into the soft tissues during an injection of local anaesthetic solution, healing may be delayed or, rarely, an abscess may form. Of a more serious nature is the possibility of the transfer of serum hepatitis which may lead to a serious and sometimes fatal illness. Apart from the risk of cross-infection, patients have a right to expect that instruments should be cleaned and sterilised before use.

STERILISATION OF INSTRUMENTS

● *Instruments penetrating soft tissues*

All instruments should be thoroughly cleaned after use and traces of blood and cement completely removed. Instruments which penetrate soft tissues, such as those used in surgical procedures, must be sterilised before use and delivered to the dentist in a sterile condition.

- *Instruments not penetrating soft tissues*

All instruments used in the mouth should be sterilised between patients but those which do not penetrate the soft tissues do not require to be delivered in a sterile but only in a clean condition. These include most conservation instruments, handpieces except those used for surgery, and suction tubes.

- *Equipment not used in the mouth*

A third group includes items of equipment not used in the mouth but which may contact the dentist's hands when he is working on a patient and could be responsible for cross-infection between patients. Examples of this group are the controls of units and the handles of triple syringes. These cannot be sterilised but should be wiped with antiseptic solution between patients.

CLEANING OF INSTRUMENTS

Instruments are usually cleaned mechanically with a small wire brush and this applies particularly to burs. Apart from the desirability of having clean instruments, cleaning before sterilising is necessary since heat sterilisation may make subsequent removal of protein more difficult. The presence of protein will reduce the bactericidal activity of the chemical disinfectants commonly used to treat burs (Neugeboren *et al.* 1972). Ultrasonic cleaners are useful but do not remove more resistant debris such as set cement or dried blood.

METHODS OF STERILISATION

Some dental hospitals operate a system of central sterilisation (Eccles 1980). After use, instruments are transported to a central area where they are sterilised and returned to the clinics. In a multiple dental practice a similar scheme may be used but in most practices instruments are sterilised in or close to the surgery.

Autoclave

The autoclave, or pressure steam steriliser, provides a rapid and

Fig. 13.1 Autoclave suitable for use in a dental practice.

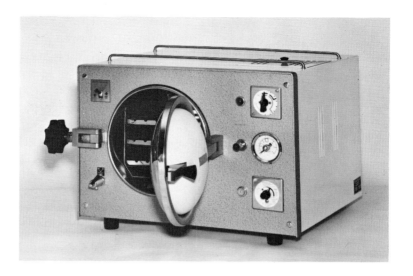

effective method of sterilising instruments, impression trays and similar pieces of equipment. Some air turbine and low-speed handpieces may be sterilised in an autoclave at temperatures up to 135°C, but only if recommended by the manufacturer and only after spraying with the recommended lubricant. For instruments which have been wrapped to ensure storage and delivery in a sterile condition, a large high-vacuum autoclave should be used. Such equipment would be available only in a hospital, but for unwrapped instruments a simple downward displacement autoclave is adequate. These are available in small sizes suitable for dental practices (Fig. 13.1). In the high-vacuum autoclave, air is first evacuated and then steam is introduced, while in the downward displacement autoclave the air is directly displaced by steam. Unwrapped instruments will be sterilised in 3 minutes at 134°C or in 15 minutes at 121°C (Rubbo & Gardner 1965). Chromium-plated steel instruments will rust if routinely autoclaved, so stainless steel is to be preferred. Where it is essential to include plated instruments, these may be wrapped in vapour phase inhibitor paper. It is most convenient to sterilise conservaton instruments in an instrument tray (Fig. 13.2). In the absence of facilities for bacteriological controls, Browne's tubes will indicate by means of a colour change that the autoclave has reached the desired temperature for an adequate time.

Dry heat steriliser

Dry heat sterilising can be used to sterilise instruments, endodon-

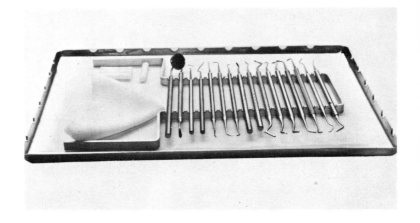

tic instruments and endodontic dressings (Fig. 13.3). A temperature of 160°C for 1 hour is adequate for sterilisation. However, this method is slow, produces excessive heat in warm weather and causes paper points to become brittle after repeated processing. Where recommended by the manufacturer some low-speed handpieces can be sterilised by dry heat up to 180°C after spraying with a special lubricant. Turbine handpieces are damaged at this temperature.

Boiling water

Boiling water is not an effective sterilising agent; boiling in water for 20 minutes will kill most bacteria but not spores or viruses. It produces excessive humidity and steam in the surgery and cannot be recommended.

Antiseptic solutions

Antiseptic solutions, such as 0.5 per cent chlorhexidine in 70 per cent alcohol, or 2 per cent glutaraldehyde solution, are useful for wiping surfaces such as controls of equipment which cannot be effectively sterilised. Dental burs should be soaked in this solution for several hours.

Disposable equipment

The use of disposable equipment has simplified some sterilisation problems. Disposable needles, sterilised by gamma radiation, are routinely used for injection of local anaesthetic solution. These are

Fig. 13.3 Dry heat steriliser.

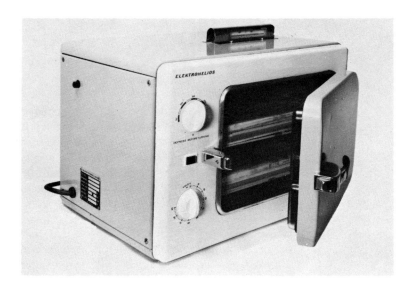

particularly valuable since it is difficult to clean the lumen of a needle effectively. The risk of fracture of such a needle is very low since it is used only once and is not subjected to high temperature. Disposable suction tubes and impression trays are available.

ASEPTIC TECHNIQUES

In operations such as the injection of local anaesthetic solution and endodontic treatment including pulp capping and surgical endodontic operations the operator must not only use sterile instruments but must also avoid contaminating them during the operation. Infection must be effectively controlled or the success of the operation may be prejudiced. While complete asepsis is desirable it is not always possible to achieve in the dental environment; nevertheless, every effort should be made to do so. The hands should be well scrubbed before commencing treatment and not contaminated by unnecessary contact with surfaces which may be infected. In endodontic treatment the teeth concerned should be free from dental plaque and isolated with rubber dam, the dam and the teeth being wiped with an antiseptic solution. Instruments should not be handled on the part which will enter the field of operation, for example the needle for injecting local anaesthetic, nor should these parts be allowed to contact unsterile surfaces before use. Used and sterile instruments should be kept apart. The assistant in the surgical operation should also have scrubbed her hands and should be adequately trained in aseptic techniques.

HYGIENE

Patients have a right to expect dentists, their staff and their surgeries to be clean and neat. It is hardly necessary to recommend frequent showers to the dentist or dental student. In hot weather the use of a deodorant spray is advisable. It is preferable for the dentist or student to change his clothing before a treatment session and to wear a shirt, trousers and shoes which have not been contaminated by everyday wear. It is also preferable for women dentists, when operating, to wear trousers since these pose fewer problems than skirts. In the absence of a complete change of clothing a protective gown is essential.

One, not uncommon, source of annoyance to patients is halitosis in a dentist. The oral hygiene of a student or dentist should be above reproach and any temporary halitosis controlled by wearing a mask. Many dentists routinely wear masks during treatment; this becomes essential when the dentist is suffering from an upper respiratory infection. The dentist's breath should not smell of tobacco or alcohol. Care of the hands and finger-nails is extremely important together with the avoidance or protection of cuts and abrasions which might act as portals for infection. Hands should be washed and scrubbed before a treatment session and washed between patients or even during treatment if they should be contaminated. A student should acquire a sense of hygiene so that during the treatment of patients his hands do not touch his face, hair or protective clothing. The use of disposable handkerchiefs is indicated.

HIGH-RISK PATIENTS

Certain patients, from whom the risk of serious infection of the dentist or other patients is high can be designated as high-risk patients. In these the normal precautions to prevent cross-infection must be considered inadequate and a very strict regimen of asepsis and antisepsis must be used (Ross & Clarke 1981; Follett & Macfarlane 1981). This may be difficult to achieve in general practice, and as a result most dental hospitals provide a service for these patients.

Hepatitis B, or serum hepatitis, is the main condition in which these special measures are required since contact with the patient's blood or saliva may lead to infection of the dentist, assistant or subsequent patients. It may be induced in patients as the result of multiple blood transfusions, even though the blood is carefully screened. It has a higher than average prevalence in patients who are receiving dialysis treatment, those who have an immunoglobulin deficiency and those suffering from leukaemia and haemophilia who may require multiple transfusions. It has been recommended that precautions should also be taken in patients suffering from Down's syndrome who live in institutions, and in drug addicts and tattooed persons where an infected needle may have been used. The blood of all such patients should be screened for the presence of Australia antigen which if positive will give an indication that they are infectious.

The dental care of such patients should be undertaken in a closed room which has been designed or modified to control the spread of infection outside the room and in which disinfection of floors, walls and work surfaces is facilitated. The treatment should be undertaken by a dentist, aided by an assistant, both of whom are aware of the risks and of the precautions which must be taken. The dentist and the assistant should wear disposable gowns, caps and gloves, with masks and visors to protect the face. Staff with abrasions on their hands or face should be excluded. Air turbines, high-speed drills with sprays, triple syringes, ultrasonic scalers and polishing techniques are all ways of spreading infection and their use should be avoided. High-volume aspirators which vent into the surgery tend to create a bacterial aerosol and should not be used, although central evacuation, venting outside the building, is satisfactory. Efficient extraction fans may be of value. Particular care must be taken with the use of needles when administering a local anaesthetic since accidental puncture of the dentist's hand after use on a patient carries a high risk of transferring the disease.

After the completion of treatment all instruments should be carefully washed, placed in a closed container and autoclaved. Impressions are soaked in a glutaraldehyde solution for 1 hour before being sent to the laboratory. The staff involved in treatment should wash their hands and faces thoroughly after the session is complete. They should report immediately to a physician if they feel unwell or if signs of jaundice appear and should be tested at intervals of 6 months for the presence of antigen in their blood.

In view of the incidence of undiagnosed hepatitis in the population it is considered advisable for dentists and assistants to routinely wear rubber gloves in procedures where their hands may be heavily contaminated by blood.

Mercury

Mercury is extensively used in dentistry in the making of amalgam restorations and should be considered a health hazard. It is a volatile liquid which, if carelessly used in a poorly ventilated surgery, may reach an atmospheric level possibly dangerous to dental personnel. Adequate ventilation of the surgery with an extractor fan will help to reduce this risk. Mixing amalgam in an amalgamator may be hazardous, particularly if the mixing capsule leaks. Using commercially capsulated amalgam, or placing the amalgamator in a cabinet with a fan to expel the air outside the building, will control this risk. An ultrasonic condenser used to pack amalgam will increase atmospheric mercury levels and should not be used (Chandler, Rupp & Paffenbarger 1971). Liquid mercury may be absorbed through cuts and abrasions and even through intact skin. Neither mercury nor unset amalgam should be touched by hand. Fragments of surplus amalgam may be swallowed if not carefully removed from the patient's mouth after a filling has been inserted. However, this appears to cause little risk to patients.

Of particular importance is the avoidance of major or minor spills of mercury. The preparation of amalgam fillings should be carried out on a special area having an impervious surface with a lipped margin and free from cracks. The floor should not be carpeted. Waste mercury and amalgam should be stored in a container, covered by a solution of potassium permanganate, and with a lid which seals the container. Particular care should be taken when loading a quantity of liquid mercury into an amalgamator and it is probably better to avoid the use of loose mercury completely and use capsulated amalgam. In the event of a major spill on the floor, expert help should be obtained and on no account should a vacuum cleaner be used.

Although mercury is a potential hazard to the dentist, reasonable precautions should be effective in avoiding this risk. The surgery should be well ventilated, capsulated amalgam should be used, the hands of all personnel mixing or using amalgam should be washed afterwards, particularly before eating and smoking. Neither of these activities should take place in the surgery. Mercury levels in hair and nails give some indication of recent exposure and if there is any suspicion that staff have been at risk, samples of these should be tested by a specialist laboratory. Atmospheric levels in the surgery can be tested with a mercury vapour meter.

Dust

Dust is produced in many dental operations. Larger particles produced in laboratory work do not reach the alveoli of the lungs but smaller particles produced during the cutting of enamel and dentine may do so. The use of suction in the mouth and the wearing of a mask by the dentist will provide some protection.

Eye damage

Damage to the eyes of the dentist or assistant may result from flying particles of tooth or filling during high-speed cutting with rotary instruments and even from fracture of tungsten carbide burs. The wearing of spectacles during cutting and polishing procedures is strongly advised.

References

CHANDLER H.H., RUPP N.W. & PAFFENBARGER G.C. (1971) *J. Amer. dent. Ass.* **82**, 553–557.

ECCLES J.D. (1980) *J. Dentistry* **8**, 3–7.

FOLLETT E.A.C. & MACFARLANE T.W. (1981) *Brit. dent. J.* **150**, 92–93.

JONES D.E. (1981) *Brit. dent. J.* **151**, 145–148.

NEUGEBOREN N., NISENGARD R.J., BEUTNER E.H. & FERGUSON G.W. (1972) *J. Amer. dent. Ass.* **85**, 123–127.

ROSS J.W. & CLARKE S.K.R. (1981) *Brit. dent. J.* **150**, 89–91.

RUBBO S.D. & GARDNER J.F. (1965) *A Review of Sterilisation and Hygiene.* Lloyd-Luke, London.

Chapter 14
Dentist–patient relationship

The success or failure of the dentist to establish the type of dental practice he wishes to have depends largely on his ability to form satisfactory professional relationships with patients. If a patient is to be encouraged to visit a dentist other than for the relief of pain, it is essential that some degree of rapport should be established. Few people view a visit to the dentist without some degree of apprehension and it is more difficult for the dentist to provide satisfactory treatment for a tense and nervous patient than for a relaxed and co-operative one, so it is in the interests of both to establish a situation whereby the patient is relaxed and the dentist can operate with freedom.

The dentist–patient relationship starts from the moment the patient enters the door of the practice and is greeted by a receptionist. If her attitude is unfriendly or brusque this is likely to increase apprehension in the patient. It is desirable to have ancillary personnel who are pleasant and understanding but who are firm when necessary. The furnishings and magazines in the waiting room should encourage patients to relax, particularly if they may have long to wait for their appointment. Long waiting periods and large numbers of patients in a waiting room are undesirable. Not only does this waste the patients' time, but the behaviour of one apprehensive patient in a waiting room can increase the level of stress in the others. Equally, the dentist will be more hurried and stressed if he is aware of a build-up of patients in the waiting area.

Once the patient enters the surgery everything must be done to give him a feeling of quiet efficiency and confidence but not of a brisk production line. Efficient treatment can be provided without giving the impression of a conveyor belt. The patient should be welcomed into the surgery by the chairside assistant, seated comfortably in the chair and a protective bib placed in position. The headrest is then adjusted so that he can feel as physically relaxed as possible.

If it is the patient's first visit, the dentist should have established beforehand from his receptionist details of the patient and the general reason for attendance. On entering the surgery he can be knowledgeable about the patient and proceed to establish precisely the patient's present problem. Having defined this, he can then take medical and dental histories. These preliminaries, if handled correctly, can establish a pleasant relationship before proceeding to an examination. A carefully conducted examination will once more give the patient an impression of thoroughness and consideration. Whenever possible it is useful to confine an initial visit to examining the patient, giving advice and cleaning the teeth. This visit should be kept fairly short thus reducing the temptation to embark on active treatment of the patient before a satisfactory relationship has been established. If the patient is in pain, relief of this will be a primary objective. The examination may then be abbreviated and attention paid to the treatment of the specific complaint.

A calm, confident manner for the dentist and freedom from pain for the patient is fundamental to a good relationship, so for subsequent visits the dentist will have planned specific treatment and decided whether a local anaesthetic will be required. Where necessary the dental surgery assistant can discreetly prepare the local anaesthetic whilst the dentist talks to the patient. Surface anaesthetic can be applied at this stage whilst the dentist explains what he is going to do during the visit. Generally, within a minute or so the patient will be reasonably relaxed and the dentist can administer the local anaesthetic. It is then essential to wait for the anaesthetic to work before starting to operate. This period can be occupied either in conversation, or in trimming and polishing the restorations placed at a previous visit.

Some patients who say that they prefer not to have a local anaesthetic because injections do not work are astounded at the freedom from pain when they are finally persuaded to have one. Frequently it is found that when they have had local anaesthetics administered previously insufficient time has been allowed for the agent to work and the whole of the cavity preparation may have been completed in the first two or three minutes before effective anaesthesia has been established. This accounts for a significant number of potentially difficult and unco-operative patients.

New patients in particular are worried and concerned about what is going to happen to them in the dentist's surgery; their fear is largely due to ignorance, and brief reassuring explanations often provide considerable relief for many apprehensive patients. It is essential at all times to be truthful with patients, but one may occasionally blur the details a little. It is a short-sighted policy to assure a patient that a potentially painful procedure will not hurt as, when a similar assurance is next offered, the patient will not be convinced. Before administering a local anaesthetic be honest with the patient and say that he may be aware of a certain amount of discomfort during the period of the injection; discomfort is a more acceptable word than pain. In certain areas where injections are particularly uncomfortable, such as in the upper anterior region, it will be necessary to tell the patient that the injection will hurt a little. It will also be necessary, when giving injections in this region, to reassure the patient that any subsequent lacrymation is a reflex reaction and not weakness of character. As time goes on and the patient realises that the dentist can be trusted to keep him informed he will become more relaxed and tolerate more extensive procedures.

The dentist must not forget the problems of patient pain just because he has given an injection of local anaesthetic. This prevents pain in a relatively localised area and other sensations than true pain can be very unpleasant for the patient. While operating the dentist must guard against extremes of pressure. It is possible to cause pain whilst supporting the mandible during the condensation of amalgam by pressing too hard into the sensitive soft tissues beneath the chin. Equally it is unpleasant for a patient if the handpiece raps sharply against the incisors as it is inserted or withdrawn from the mouth. Similar problems may be produced by the vibration of certain cutting and condensing instruments or an inappropriately positioned suction tube.

The problem of after-pain is rather different but equally important. The soft tissues within the area of anaesthesia can be maltreated during an operation without the knowledge of the patient. When the anaesthesia wears off the patient will be fully aware of any cuts, abrasions or bruising which have been produced. Clearly the anaesthetised soft tissues should be handled as gently as the unanaesthetised ones if these are to be minimised. Lastly, when superficial anaesthesia is likely to be prolonged much beyond the end of the appointment, the patient should be warned of the risks of burning or biting their tissues. Thoughtfulness and consideration over these matters takes little time and helps to convince the patient that the dentist is actively interested in his welfare. This, in turn, encourage greater co-operation in achieving good oral hygiene and the practice of other preventive measures such as diet control.

The above remarks represent one simple approach to the dentist–patient relationship. It is impossible, however, to provide detailed instruction on how an individual dentist may establish a satisfactory relationship with any individual patient. The precise form and manner of dentist–patient relationships will inevitably vary with both the style and character of the dentist and patient, but many of the components are well discussed by Samson (1969). The basic ingredients of the relationship are trust, freedom from pain and freedom from apprehension. In the average patient apprehension will be sufficiently controlled by the knowledge that the procedures will be relatively painless and the technique of atraumatically administering a local anaesthetic is therefore discussed. In the abnormally apprehensive patient this is, in itself, not enough and it is necessary, therefore, to consider other methods of relieving pain and apprehension such as general anaesthesia and sedation.

Local anaesthesia

The safest and most generally satisfactory method of achieving this objective is by the use of a local anaesthetic. Unfortunately, there is a widespread fear of injections and this has to be overcome if progress is to be made. This fear may be associated with early childhood experiences of intramuscular injections of antibiotics or diphtheria immunisation, but a significant number of people have been adversely affected by careless dental local anaesthetic technique and it is therefore pertinent to consider some of the basic procedures involved in the administration of a dental local anaesthetic.

- Explain to the patient where the injection is to be administered and the degree of discomfort to be anticipated.
- Carefully dry the area to be injected and apply surface anaesthetic and antiseptic if desired.
- Collect the syringe from the assistant. Working outside the patient's line of vision and using an aseptic technique, the assistant will have fitted the sterile hypodermic syringe with a disposable needle and inserted a cartridge of local anaesthetic solution. The solution should have been pre-heated to body temperature to reduce the discomfort of the injection.
- Gently stretch the mucosa through which the needle is to pass, as penetration occurs more smoothly and comfortably through taut tissue.
- Bring the syringe into position and penetrate the mucosa. The movements leading up to this should be carried out carefully and the patient should not be startled by rapid movements or the thoughtless waving of the syringe in front of his face. It is useful if at this stage the dentist can maintain a steady flow of conversation and 'talk the patient through the injection'.

- Apply light pressure to the plunger of the syringe as soon as the needle is in the tissues so that very small quantities of solution are ejected ahead of the needle.
- Advance the needle slowly into the tissues behind this 'shield' of anaesthetic solution and when the tip has reached the required position, deposit the appropriate amount of solution slowly and gently into the tissues. Too rapid deposition of fluid produces pain at the time of injection and can lead to post-operative discomfort from bruising of the tissues. Where practicable, aspiration prior to injection is desirable to ensure that the local anaesthetic is not being deposited in a blood vessel.
- Remove the needle neatly from the tissues and return the syringe to the assistant or place it on one side out of the patient's line of vision.

Surface anaesthesia This is achieved by the application of creams or sprays to the dry mucosa before the injection is given. If a suitable period of time is allowed to elapse after application, anaesthesia of the superficial tissues will be produced so that the patient does not feel the initial entry of the needle. These agents do not, however, prevent discomfort from the passage of the needle into the deeper tissues or the sensation associated with the discharge of the local anaesthetic solution. The effective application of these agents also requires a patient to sit for a period waiting for surface anaesthesia to develop. The individual dentist must decide the relative importance of these factors and the decision whether or not to use a surface anaesthetic will vary from dentist to dentist and possibly also from patient to patient.

APPREHENSIVE PATIENTS

Many dental patients are apprehensive to some degree but are able to accept treatment in the normal way if the dentist shows patience and understanding and avoids painful or traumatic experiences. However, a small proportion of patients are apprehensive to the extent where they pose a difficult problem to the dentist in the provision of dental care. In these cases a two-fold approach should be used: the use of considerable patience and understanding, and the use of drugs.

With a very apprehensive patient the dentist should take several short visits to assess the degree of apprehension and the type of measure required. The usual stages are:

- Encourage the patient to sit in the dental chair.

- Carry out an examination without instruments.
- Use a mirror to examine the teeth.
- Use a soft rubber cup to polish the teeth.
- Examine by means of a probe.
- Administer a local anaesthetic in an area where injection can be relatively painless, for example the buccal sulcus opposite the upper molar teeth.
- Prepare a small cavity.

Gradation of approach and treatment of this nature will be successful with many patients. However, in a small proportion of cases this approach will not be successful and the dentist may have to think in terms of sedation or general anaesthesia.

Sedation

The number of patients for whom this is essential is small (Curson & Coplans 1970) and the liberal use of sedation for the ambulant patient is sometimes a substitute for satisfactory patient management. The sedated patient is conscious, requires a local anaesthetic and can co-operate to some degree with the dentist. It follows that sedation is not suitable for the very unco-operative patient. Sedatives are normally administered by one of three routes, orally, intravenously or by inhalation.

Oral

The most commonly used tranquilliser is diazepam. The effect of this when administered orally to patients receiving dental treatment is frequently unsatisfactory owing to delayed or irregular absorption. In moderately apprehensive patients it may be useful if it is felt that the taking of a pill would be of psychological value. However, where management problems are so severe that effective sedation is considered essential the intravenous or inhalational routes are indicated.

Intravenous

Diazepam is now the recommended drug. With this there is little risk of producing unconsciousness but there is a risk of irritation to the veins close to the site of injection. However, this technique carries a greater risk than working on a normal patient and should not be undertaken without all the necessary equipment to deal with emergencies which may arise, or without an adequate complement of trained personnel.

Inhalation

The use of a preset mixture of oxygen air and 25 per cent nitrous oxide has been described (Edmunds & Rosen 1975, 1983). Techniques of this type which offer effective sedation without risk of producing loss of consciousness or eliminating the cough reflex have been accepted as suitable for use by dentists in conventional surgery conditions without a second qualified doctor or dentist in attendance. Techniques which involve the regulation of the concentrations of gases by the dentist, and where the level of nitrous oxide can exceed 30 per cent are more appropriately categorised as general anaesthetics and a second trained clinician must be present (Seward *et al.* 1981).

General anaesthesia

There is a very small group of patients for whom conservation under general anaesthesia is essential due to the severe behavioural problems or some local or systemic condition. The duration of the anaesthetic required for routine conservation is relatively long and the remarks made in relation to intravenous sedation apply equally to this situation. It is the opinion of the authors that conservation under general anaesthesia purely on the grounds of patient preference is undesirable and should be discouraged.

Hypnosis

This is a very specialised field in which few people have extensive experience. There is no doubt that in some patients dramatic results can be produced using hypnosis either to reinforce local anaesthesia or even in the absence of conventional anaesthesia, and this is a field worthy of further investigation.

References

Curson I. & Coplans M.P. (1970) *Brit. dent. J.* **128**, 19–22.
Edmunds D.H. & Rosen M. (1975) *Brit. dent. J.* **139**, 398–402.
Edmunds D.H. & Rosen M. (1983) *Dental Update*, In press.
Samson E. (1969) *The Management of Dental Practice*, Chs 6 and 7. Kimpton, London.
Seward G.R., Bramley P., Vickers M.D.A., Fordyce G.L. & Dinsdale R.C.W. (1981) *Brit. dent. J.* **151**, 390–391.

Index